BARAGWANATH HOSPITAL, SOWETO
A HISTORY OF MEDICAL CARE 1941–1990

T0355639

BARAGWANATH HOSPITAL, Soweto

A history of medical care 1941–1990

SIMONNE HORWITZ

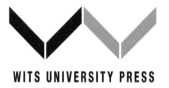

WITS UNIVERSITY PRESS

Published in South Africa by:
Wits University Press
1 Jan Smuts Avenue
Johannesburg

www.witspress.co.za

First published 2013

ISBN 978-1-86814-747-2 (print)
ISBN 978-1-86814-748-9 (digital)

Cover photograph and Plate 7 copyright ©David Goldblatt
Cover design by Hothouse South Africa
Design and layout by Sheaf Publishing, Benoni
Printed and bound by Paarlmedia, Paarl

Contents

Acknowledgements

Baragwanath Hospital is an intimidating institution. I remember driving past it on numerous trips to Soweto, and its size, organisational complexity and the social milieu in which it is set were overwhelming – and yet fascinating. In distilling such complexity into this book I owe debts of gratitude over three continents.

Of course, my largest debt of gratitude is to the remarkable women and men who worked at Baragwanath Hospital over the years. In 2004 they welcomed me into their homes, offices and wards; they wrote me letters, shared memories, photos and personal papers; they tried to educate me in the 'Bara ways'. I hope that I have done some justice to their words, dedication, knowledge and experiences. Their names are reflected in the text, but I want to point, in particular, to those with whom I spoke in the course of interviews which took place in 2004 and 2005.

In South Africa I want to thank June Gerrard, who first inspired my love of history at high school, as well as the incredible teachers Sue Jordaan and Cherie Robinson, who taught me to write and construct an argument. At the University of the Witwatersrand (Wits) I was fortunate enough to be taught, advised and inspired by an exceptional group of Africanists who laid the ground on which this book was built. In particular, I should like to thank Philip Bonner, David Coplan, Clive Glaser, Isabel Hofmeyr, Deborah James and Isak 'Sakkie' Niehaus. Peter Delius first encouraged me to do graduate work and then talked through and advised on many aspects of the project, remaining a teacher, mentor and friend to whom I owe much. Emily Craven, Sarah Kashula, Chris Malaudzi and Linn Hjort embarked on the postgraduate journey with me and provided support, friendship, challenging questions, proofreading, translations, and biscuits.

For access to resources at the Wits Faculty of Health Sciences I should like to thank Max Price. Rochelle Keene and Cheryl-Anne Comrie of the Adler Museum of Medicine who provided access to material and support and help on this and other projects. My thanks are also due to Carol Archibald at Wits Historical Papers, Zofia Sulej of the Wits Central Archives, Rowena Wilkinson at the Military History Museum and the staff at the National Archives in Pretoria. The William Cullen Library at Wits has, since my time as an undergraduate, been a place of discovery for me and its fascinating and extensive Africana collection has shaped my understanding of South African history. The Africana librarians, Margaret Northey and Fay Blain, two of the most professional, kind and knowledgeable librarians I have met – deserve many thanks. Mercy Kgarume, Sophie Motsewabone and Rachel Louis from Government Publications retrieved numerous volumes from the dusty basement for me over the years.

In Oxford, St Antony's College offered not only a physical, but also one of the finest intellectual homes one could wish for. My college proved to be an environment in which I could learn, explore and grow, and for that I will be forever grateful. My Oxford friends are credited with keeping me well-balanced, teaching me so much and sharing this journey with me, even as we dispersed all over the world. I want to thank especially Mark Abrahamson, Chris Andreas, Annelies Blom, Julian Brown, Karen Brown, Nicole Evans, Patrick Fothergill, Niharika Gupta, Rebecca Hodes, Sonja Keller, Amna Khalid, Rebekah Lee, Sloan Mahone, Harriet Nuwagaba, Paul Ocobock, Paul Petzschmann and Krista Zongolowicz.

Dwight Newman's support, encouragement and belief in my ability to complete this project were vital, as was his practical assistance. He challenged my views and made me clarify my arguments. My history methodology relied on his height, which enabled physical access to sources stored out of my reach on top shelves of storerooms at Baragwanath, and he proofread and edited every word of the thesis.

Professors Shula Marks and Megan Vaughan have long served as academic role models. It was in the UK that I got to know both. Shula's work has inspired much of what I have done and her interest in my project, her encouragement and the invitations to celebrate festivals with her family when I was lonely and far from home will forever be appreciated. From the time I first took Megan's class during my Master's, right through to the end of this project, she has encouraged me to read and think outside of my comfort zone. As a supervisor Megan never lost sight of the big picture and arguments, even when I wanted to focus more and more narrowly. Her challenging questions, guidance and support have meant so much to me. Even after she moved to Cambridge, Megan kept me on as a student, and for that I am most grateful.

Our meetings, often over coffee at the British Library, re-enthused me and always gave me a renewed confidence in my work.

During my time in Oxford I was privileged to be part of an exciting and innovative group of students and researchers who gathered around Professor William Beinart and who made a rich and rewarding environment in which to work. As a supervisor, William guided the thesis and its author with remarkable insight, patience and knowledge. He was realistic even when I was not, and his supervision and personal support have been invaluable. As a scholar, supervisor and person, William has always motivated and inspired me and I benefited hugely from being his student.

I have a number of organisations to thank for financial support. It was a Rhodes Scholarship that first saw me on the path to Oxford. The Rhodes Trust provided not only the financial support for my Master's and first two years of my D.Phil but also an international community of friends and colleagues. I am indebted to the Skye Foundation for their year of funding and also for their inspiring approach to education. In my final year I was supported by my alma mater through the Wits Overseas Scholarship, and I am grateful that they saw the value in my project and continue to support alumni. For research funding I wish to thank St Antony's College, the Collin Mathews Fund, Commonwealth Fund and the Wingate Scholarship.

The process of turning the thesis into this book took place at the University of Saskatchewan in Canada. Professor Jim Miller and his Canada Research Chair offered me a physical and intellectual space to work on the transformation. His guidance, support and advice are much appreciated. Also at the University of Saskatchewan I should like to thank Jim Handy, Bob Stock, Lisa Smith and Mark Meyers for engaging in my work, and offer particular thanks to Erika Dyck and Valerie Korinek. Erika and Valerie became my cheerleading team in the final stages of this project; they read and commented on chapters, advised and shared their experiences willingly and kindly to the real benefit of this book and its author, all the while learning more about Baragwanath Hospital than they probably ever wanted to know.

It is fitting that this book be published by Wits University Press and I should like to thank the team there: Roshan Cader, Melanie Pequeux, Corina van der Spoel, Veronica Klipp and especially to my fantastic and engaged editor, Monica Seeber.

Finally, my most important thanks are to my sibling Leanne, also a historian and extraordinary teacher, and to my parents, Dawn and Lewis. My parents believed in the absolute value of education and supported my studies in every way. Throughout my academic career my mother has proofread my essays and my father helped me gather information, photographed it, drove me to appointments and helped in every way possible. I hope they know how much their practical help has contributed to this work, but most importantly my parents have continued to love, feed and support me. They put up with the visits home which were more research trips than visits and with my constant refrain that I was 'almost finished'. My dad passed away before he saw the transformation of the thesis into this book, and although his passing leaves a huge hole in all of our lives I think he would be very happy that this project is finally finished.

This book is dedicated to my parents and to all those whose lives have been touched, shaped and affected by what goes on within the walls of Chris Hani Baragwanath Hospital.

List of Illustrations

Plate 1: Early aerial photograph of Baragwanath as a military hospital. Courtesy the author.

Plate 2: Premature baby unit (Ward 40) at Baragwanath Hospital in the 1950s being heated by a coal-fired tubular stoves. Photograph by Professor Sam Wayburne.

Plate 3: Outpatients ward in the 1950s. Courtesy MuseumAfrica.

Plate 4: Patients on mattresses being tended by nurses and doctors. Courtesy MuseumAfrica.

Plate 5: Aerial photograph of Baragwanath Hospital with Soweto in the background. Courtesy the author.

Plate 6: Nurses' strike at Baragwanath Hospital in the late 1950s. Courtesy MuseumAfrica.

Plate 7: Mothers watching over babies on drips being treated for gastroenteritis. Photograph by David Goldblatt.

Plate 8: Nurses treating patients in post-operative care. Photograph by Claude Provost, *Panorama Magazine* 1967

List of Abbreviations

Adler Museum	Adler Museum of the History of Medicine, Wits University
Bara PR Archives	Baragwanath Public Relations Department Archives
BHBM	Baragwanath Hospital Board Minutes
DMF	Department of Medicine Files and Archives
GES	Gesondheid – Department of Health, Pretoria
HBR	Hospital Secretary, Hospital Board Records
IRC	University of the Witwatersrand, Faculty of Health Sciences, Internal Reconciliation Commission
JHM	Johannesburg Hospital: Medical Superintendent Files Archive
Medunsa	Medical University of South Africa
NTS	Archive of the Secretary of Native Affairs
PRO	Public Relations Office
PWD	Public Works Department
SAB	Central Archive Depot, Pretoria National Archive
SADF	South African Defence Force
SAMDC	South African Medical and Dental Council
SAMJ	South African Medical Journal
SANA	South African Nursing Association
SANC	South African Nursing Council
TPA	Transvaal Provincial Administration
TRC	Truth and Reconciliation Commission
UDF	United Democratic Front
VdH Papers	Chris van den Heever Personal Papers
WHP	University of the Witwatersrand, Department of Historical Papers
WHSL	University of the Witwatersrand, Health Sciences Library
WHSR	University of the Witwatersrand, Faculty of Health Science Registry Archives
WISER	Wits Institute of Social and Economic Research
Wits Archives	University of the Witwatersrand Central Archives and Registry
Wits	University of the Witwatersrand

A note on terminology

This book is as much a history of one specific hospital as it is a history of medicine in the apartheid state. As such, the use of racial terminology is both unavoidable and important in showing the very nature of apartheid thinking and the social, economic and political implications of the ways in which these terms were employed. In this book the labels 'African', 'white', 'coloured' and 'Indian' are used as they are widely understood in South Africa today. The term 'black' is also used to refer to 'African', 'coloured' and 'Indian' people together. In historical context the terms such as 'Native', 'Bantu', 'European' and 'Non-European' are also used when citing documents or labels developed at the time.

CHAPTER 1

Introduction
A Hospital in Soweto

Intake night – Baragwanath Hospital[1]

Mbuyiseni Oswald Mtshali

The ward was like a battlefield –
victims of war
waged in the dark alley
flocked in cars, taxis, ambulances, vans and trucks.

They bore
knife wounds
axe wounds
bullet wounds
burns and lacerations.

A stench
of fresh blood
warm urine
excreta,
mingled with iodine and methylated spirits.

Groans
sighs
moans – Help me doctor!
curses – C'mon bloody nurse!

Doctors darting
from place to place
with harried nurses at their sides.

'So! It's Friday night!
Everybody is enjoying
in Soweto.'

Baragwanath Hospital[2]

Oupa Thando Mthimkulu

Speak Baragwanath speak
How many souls did you swallow
Who were intentionally killed
Who genuinely and sincerely died
How many arrived satisfactorily dead
Come Bara, tell us the real tale
Of your patients – what do you have to say?

Are they really gone forever
Did they all have inquests
Did they all claim indemnities
How many won their cases
Baragwanath hospital, big one
Are you hospitable enough
To testify to us all?

Baragwanath Hospital was built on the outskirts of the burgeoning black township that would become Soweto, situated just over twenty kilometres from Johannesburg, South Africa's wealthiest and most populous city – not only the largest hospital serving black Africans in South Africa but also the largest specialist hospital in the southern hemisphere (the hospital's size was recognised in the *Guinness Book of Records* in 1997). Over its lifespan, Baragwanath has gained a legendary status. The Soweto tourist industry includes 'Bara' – as the hospital has come to be affectionately known – as a highlight of the 'Day-in-Soweto' tours. Many medical students and doctors from around the world have passed through the hospital for their dose of the 'Bara experience' – considered unique because of the sheer numbers of patients, the severity of the pathology presented, and the quantity of trauma cases treated. Baragwanath was (and is) ever-present in the media. In the popular imagination and in official publications the hospital's distinctiveness has often been invoked:

> Baragwanath Hospital is unique – it is unique in its size (3 000 beds); it is unique in the variety and quantity of medical conditions seen; it is unique in its blend of so-called first and third-world medicine; it is unique in its witnessing of the transition of a population from a rural to an urban existence.[3]

At the same time, Baragwanath has also held a special place in apartheid South Africa, and its rich and contradictory history gives a unique insight into the inner workings of apartheid health care.

Many people in South Africa and in the broader medical community have heard about the hospital and know something of its legacy but it has not been the subject of extended historical study. Aside from reminiscences by medical staff, little has been written about the institution, the types of services it has provided or how these changed over the apartheid period. We know very little about those who worked in Baragwanath's wards and corridors, how they viewed the hospital, and the way they sought to project their views and experiences. Little is known about the institutional dynamics of the hospital or how these were shaped by the broader social and political context.

This book aims to illustrate how this rapidly growing, underfunded but surprisingly effective institution found the niche that allowed it to exist, to provide medical care to a massive patient body and at times even to flourish in the apartheid state. Baragwanath's story is the narrative of an institution within the apartheid structures that did not always function in ways that we might expect it to function. Baragwanath's history offers new ways of exploring the history of apartheid and, more specifically, of apartheid medicine and health care.

Every aspect of Baragwanath's long history has been shaped by a complex set of conditions. Its establishment in the early 1940s was no exception. Baragwanath Hospital stands on land purchased by the Cornish immigrant

John Albert Baragwanath during the late nineteenth century. He arrived in South Africa in 1886 and sought riches through a number of ventures, one of which was to purchase a site that was one day's journey by ox-wagon from Johannesburg, at the point where the road to Kimberley joined the road from Vereeniging. Here he set up a refreshment post, trading store and hotel. The hotel was known officially as the Junction Hotel and later the Wayside Inn, but to the transport drivers and their passengers who visited it, it was known as 'Baragwanath's Place' or just 'Baragwanath',[4] and the land around the hotel also became known as 'Baragwanath' (the surname is Welsh, from *bara* meaning bread and *gwenith* meaning wheat). In the early twentieth century, Baragwanath's land was bought by the Corner House Mining Group and later taken over by Crown Mines Ltd, but it was never mined. As is described in Chapter 2, the British government bought the land in the early 1940s in order to build a military hospital – and apart from his name, the only other memorial to John Albert Baragwanath is the lectern in the chapel of St Luke that is part of the Baragwanath complex.

Dr Chris van den Heever, whose involvement with Baragwanath Hospital stretched over more than three decades and who retired as chief superintendent of the hospital in the late 1990s, uses the metaphor of the phoenix, ancient symbol of rebirth, immortality and renewal shown on the hospital's coat of arms, to characterise the hospital's transformations; when the phoenix neared the end of its life it ignited itself and was reduced to ashes, and from the ashes a new phoenix was born.

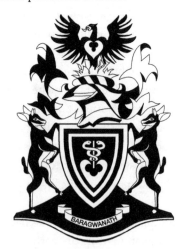

Figure 1: The Baragwanath coat of arms

By 1947 the 'phoenix' of Baragwanath as a military hospital had died but in 1948, under the auspices of the Transvaal Provincial Administration (TPA), a civilian 'phoenix' arose. In this incarnation the hospital opened with 480 beds and, as will be discussed in Chapter 2, its first patients were transferred from the non-European wing of the Johannesburg General Hospital in the 'white' area of Johannesburg. Administratively, Baragwanath became part of the Johannesburg General Hospital. Links were immediately forged between the University of the Witwatersrand (Wits) and Baragwanath which would, over the following decades, become one of its largest teaching centres. The links between the university and the hospital, as Chapter 3 shows, affected the hospital's character and capacity to provide effective medical care – but also brought medical students and their teachers into direct contact with apartheid in the medical sphere.

The 'phoenix' of the civilian hospital came of age in an increasingly racially segregated South Africa. Every aspect of the hospital was segregated. Doctors' eating, sleeping and tea facilities were separate. Black doctors and students were made to use prefabricated buildings that compared unfavourably to the facilities for whites. Doctors' salaries were determined by race and were, in general, vastly unequal. Even the rationale behind some of the building expansion at the hospital was fundamentally rooted in apartheid logic: for example, the establishment of a maternity ward in the late 1960s had as much to do with the government's desire to prevent black women giving birth at the Bridgman Memorial Hospital in 'white Johannesburg' as it did with the needs of the Soweto population. The state feared that an increasing number of black children born at Bridgman might claim rights under section 10 of the Group Areas Act to remain in Johannesburg.[5]

Baragwanath's location on the outskirts of Soweto, the heart of the anti-apartheid resistance movement, meant that medical staff cared for the victims and subjects of the apartheid state on a daily basis and the hospital was at the centre of a number of critical turning points in the struggle against apartheid. The 1955 Congress of the People and the adoption of the Freedom Charter happened in the shadows of the hospital. It was to Baragwanath that those who were shot in the back during the Sharpeville Massacre of 1960 (when police opened fire on about 5 000 Africans peacefully protesting the system of pass laws – 69 were killed and 180 wounded, most shot in the back while fleeing from the police) were transferred. On 16 June 1976, about 15 000 students from Soweto schools staged a protest march against the conditions imposed on them by Bantu Education, most notably the introduction of Afrikaans as the medium of instruction. When police opened fire one of the first victims was thirteen-year-old Hector Pieterson. Sam Nzima's photograph of the dying Pieterson being carried by another student has become an iconic image of the anti-apartheid struggle. From the time Hector Pieterson's body was transferred from Phomolong Clinic to the hospital, and during the violence that followed, Baragwanath was embroiled in an event that not only changed the history of South Africa but also had a significant effect on the hospital as discussed (with specific reference to the core medical personnel) in Chapters 4 and 5. As the violence mounted during the late 1970s and into the 1980s, Baragwanath tried to patch up and heal the broken bodies. Its doctors and nurses witnessed and responded to the changing patterns of violence as the weapons of choice in the township shifted from bicycle spokes and knives to guns.

Baragwanath also treated individuals whose illnesses were an indirect result of the policies of the apartheid state: patients suffering from the diseases associated with rapid urbanisation, inadequate housing and poor sanitation. It treated sexually transmitted diseases as well as the effects of alcoholism and violence that were by-products of the breakdown of social relationships.

Yet this was also a time when Baragwanath Hospital made some rather remarkable achievements. By 1953 the hospital had grown into an institution with 1 600 beds. In the same year, an autonomous board was appointed, allowing the hospital to operate independently from Johannesburg Hospital. By the end of the decade, Baragwanath served as one of the major centres of biomedicine in southern Africa. In the words of the second superintendent, Isadore Frack, the hospital's vital statistics:

> ... are themselves breathtaking and startling – 1 600 beds soon to be increased by a further 740; close on half-a-million outpatients annually; over 160 full-time doctors half of whom are specialists, while the other half are being trained to become specialists; over 800 nurses, 230 of whom are qualified; an annual expenditure exceeding £1 500 000 excluding capital costs; forty-six wards; ten of the most modern and best equipped surgical theatres in the country; the building of six and the taking over of a further eight peripheral municipal clinics; these represent only the bare bones of our story.[6]

In many cases the way staff treated and interacted with the patients and community around the hospital showed the scope that Baragwanath opened up for progressive activities and actions – which complicates the standard views of apartheid institutions and the delivery of health care in those times. In her influential book *The Making of Apartheid*, Deborah Posel argues that there was no all-encompassing, preconceived 'grand design' in the implementation of apartheid but that apartheid's policies were constantly being contested and reshaped by internal and external factors.[7] I argue that institutions such as Baragwanath Hospital, which grew up in the apartheid era, were, similarly, never under the hegemonic control of the apartheid system. Even under the omnipresent gaze of the state, individuals retained agency, and contested spaces opened up in ways which challenged apartheid's supremacy.

Despite government's pumping more money into health care for blacks as part of a series of more general reforms of the 1980s, Baragwanath faced increased pressure on several fronts. The overcrowding was becoming unbearable and the wards were chronically understaffed and underfunded. In the late 1980s Baragwanath suffered a series of crippling strikes. The hospital was not spared the increasing labour tensions, violence and effects of inequality that plagued the rest of the country.

In 1990, when the hospital system underwent some significant changes, another phoenix died. In the early 1990s South Africa was moving towards liberation. The National Party, unable to quell the violent opposition which festered from the mid-1970s, began to repeal discriminatory legislation. There were also significant shifts in health care. Spurred on by the glimpses of reform, progressive groups intensified the campaign for community oriented primary health care (PHC) to be a central pillar of any new health care system. This aspiration was initially outlined by a group of young liberals whose influence shaped the vision of a new medical era outlined in the South African Health Services Commission of 1942–44.[8] The Health Services Commission Report ultimately rejected hospital-based care as the core element of health service provision in South Africa, arguing for an extension of community health care projects such as that which Sidney and Emily Kark had established at Pholela in Natal in the late 1930s. But the community-oriented health initiative was short-lived. After the National Party came to power in 1948, the system was abandoned, primarily through financial strangulation by a government increasingly focused on curative care. However, the ideas of social medicine did not fade. The Freedom Charter, the statement of core principles adopted by anti-apartheid organisations at the Congress of the People in 1955, called for a preventive health care scheme run by the state as well as free medical care, with special care for mothers and children.

By the late 1970s, doctors who opposed apartheid were increasingly disillusioned with the Medical Association of South Africa (MASA) and the South African Medical and Dental Council (SAMDC). The former, the major organisational and representative body of South African doctors, became increasingly supportive of and complicit in the state's policy of separate development, whereas the latter had been formed in 1829, initially to register medical personnel and later to regulate the conduct of health professionals and to oversee standards of practice and training. From the 1970s it comprised thirty-four members, most of whom were appointed by the minister of health and thus owed their allegiance to the state. In 1982 the more racially inclusive and politically diverse National Medical and Dental Association (NAMDA) was formed as an alternative to these bodies; it took a strong stand against apartheid and also saw PHC as a guiding principle. In 1987, NAMDA formed the Progressive Primary Health Care (PPHC) network.

It was in this context and at the same time that the National Policy for Health Act, 116 of 1990 and the National Health Service Delivery Plan 1991 aimed to made far-reaching changes to health and hospital administration.[9] This new legislation centralised control of the health care system and budget under the national minister and shifted the emphasis to primary health care. The heads of major tertiary hospitals such as Baragwanath resisted the shift of funding from their hospitals to local authorities. This was not the only opposition to the changes; local-level health authorities declared the legislation unconstitutional and the African National Congress (ANC) campaigned against 'unilateral restructuring' during the period of negotiations towards national democratic elections. At the same time, Rina Venter, the minister of national health and population development, announced the desegregation, at least in theory, of thirty hospitals.

Writing in 1993, Van den Heever was certain that as the country moved towards democracy a new phoenix would again arise and bring health care to a liberated South African population. To some degree his vision has been fulfilled. The hospital now serves a democratic South Africa in which the Bill of Rights in the Constitution states that everyone has the right to access health care services. As part of the transformation the hospital has been renamed Chris Hani Baragwanath, after the slain ANC leader and *Umkhonto we Sizwe* (MK) activist. Yet, the hospital still faces the mammoth challenges of chronic underfunding, overcrowding, demoralised staff and the horrors of the HIV/AIDS pandemic.

As the country continues to grapple with these issues, it is vital to understand not only the structural inequalities that underlie the health care system, but also the history of the specific institutions. This is particularly true for the major state hospitals like Baragwanath that have formed a key element of the health care system. This history fills some of the gaps in the record. It focuses on the establishment of the hospital and provides an insight into its complex and contradictory life. It contains the experiences and views of the two professional groups (doctors and nurses) whose views of themselves, and interaction with the hospital and broader political context, shaped Baragwanath's institutional logic and ethos. The 'Bara ethos', although difficult to define, seems to have been centred on a dedication to the hospital, an unfailing belief in the importance of the medicine practised there and the ability of the Baragwanath staff to cope with and even thrive on the difficult work and huge patient load. The 'Bara ethos' included a commitment and loyalty to the hospital and fellow staff. These ideas created and reinforced the mythical status that Baragwanath developed.

Carrying out a history of Baragwanath Hospital

Driving along the Old Potchefstroon Road, the main thoroughfare between Johannesburg and Soweto, it is impossible to miss the gigantic structures that make up the hospital complex. Almost everyone in Soweto has a 'Bara' story and the hospital looms large in the medical history of South Africa even though patients, visitors, doctors and nurses were often repulsed by the conditions they saw in the wards and the conditions under which they worked. Surely, I thought, as I embarked on this study, there must be a detailed history of this remarkable hospital and its place in apartheid South Africa. There was not.

Until the mid-twentieth century, literature on 'the hospital' in the history of medicine has largely been concerned with institutional changes from pre-enlightenment charitable homes for the sick poor, often with a religious association, to secular technological institutions at the centre of medical learning. For some, such as Foucault, the turning point in the way the hospital was utilised and viewed came with the French Revolution at the end of the eighteenth century; medicine changed radically, entering, taking over and dramatically altering the hospital, and practical clinical training replaced book-based education as the centre of medical education.[10] This version of the development of the hospital is not universally accepted, however, and other historians have suggested that change happened more slowly, over a longer period.[11]

Despite contested analyses of change, historians have seen the twentieth-century hospital as the centre of both curative practices and research, directed by a bureaucracy of official administrators as well as physicians. The latter, armed with what has been called an 'intimidating arsenal of tools and techniques', increasingly dominated the medical institutions.[12] Physicians used specialist knowledge to control not only members of the medical profession but also many other aspects in their sphere of influence. Many of these early studies, written by academics and by medical personnel, focused on practitioners and their role in changing medical developments. In these analyses the hospital was at the centre of professionalised medicine but tended to be depicted as existing in relative isolation from society.[13]

In the late 1970s and 1980s such analyses, emphasising the central place of specialist hospitals in biomedicine, came under criticism – especially in the United States. There, hospitals were increasingly seen as an instrument of class and sexual oppression, where white, predominantly male, doctors came to control the medical marketplace. At the same time, academic discussions of the hospital began to consider the question of bureaucratic control. Studies considering these themes developed a far more complex understanding than could emerge from a narrative of medical developments alone.[14] Increasingly, these studies focused on the hospital's interactions with external forces and non-medical staff. Their social and geographical origins, expectations, relationship to patients and the administration, the nature of their work and their perspectives on what transpires within the hospital are all seen as part of the legitimate social history of the hospital, and reflect broader social divisions of race and gender. These are histories that seek to place the hospital in its social, political and geographic context.

This book draws on such insights but expands on the approach by providing a microanalysis of an institution and its staff which allows for the development of an in-depth understanding of how the broader context shaped the functioning of the institution and also the experience of those who worked within it, particularly the doctors and nurses.

Much of the groundbreaking general work on the history of the hospitals in the United States and Britain seems to have occurred during the 1980s, with fewer studies produced during the next decade. One significant study from the later period, and which has influenced my work, is Guenter Risse's *Mending Bodies, Saving Souls*. It echoes earlier concerns about the changing nature of the hospital, but takes a different approach from many of its predecessors, offering a history through a series of what the author calls 'hospital narratives and case studies'.[15] Through these vignettes, the author presents a more nuanced and vibrant study than those which paint institutional transformations in broad strokes. I too have tried to use specific occurrences at Baragwanath, and the detailed life stories of hospital administrators, doctors and nurses, to present a vivid, nuanced and individualised account of the history of Baragwanath Hospital.

Many of the prominent studies of the hospital in history have been broad-based rather than focused on individual institutions. The majority of single institution studies have been written in-house, or as commissioned histories under the auspices of the institution involved, and tend to ignore the individual hospital's social context.[16] They confine their scope to the development of the hospital in terms of the medical achievements of the clinicians, the physical construction of the hospital, and a triumphalist account of the services offered. The nurses are often absent (except as helpers of the clinicians) from these histories, which do not take us inside the hospital. My approach builds on studies integrating social context into the analysis, but also highlights the social dynamics of a single institution, attempting to capture some of its characteristics, conflicts and ethos through individual experiences.

Histories of medicine and hospitals in South Africa have tended to fall into two main groups. The first consists of general studies which have focused on the introduction of Western medicine to South Africa and on the medical conquest of disease.[17] More recently, medical institutions, and especially specialist hospitals such as leprosaria, psychiatric hospitals or disease-specific institutions have begun to gain academic attention. The only significant general hospital history in South Africa is the recently published multiauthor history of Groote Schuur Hospital in Cape Town, a book that offers a complex, multifaceted history – but the story of Groote Schuur is very different to that of Baragwanath. Groote Schuur was a hospital with a singular regional history and it was located far more centrally and was as much part of the University of Cape Town Medical School complex as the Johannesburg Hospital was part of the Wits complex. Baragwanath, on the other hand, was situated a long drive from central Johannesburg in the heart of the black township of Soweto. Another significant difference between Baragwanath and Groote Schuur was that the latter has always been a hospital serving both black and white patients (although segregated during the apartheid era).[18] If we are to understand the complexity of apartheid health and medicine it is important to hear the multiple voices of those who worked within the broad spectrum of health care delivery, and the voices of those who worked at Baragwanath though all its incarnations are a significant part of this understanding.

Yet the only existing discussions of Baragwanath's history fit into the second category of writing on the history of hospitals in South Africa which include popular accounts, personal narratives and histories of individual hospitals written predominantly by insiders and consisting of personal reminiscences, or in celebration of centenaries. These works often present hospitals in relative isolation from social forces and tend to focus on medical and scientific developments. They do, of course, provide useful first-hand accounts of individual experiences and medical developments within a range of hospitals.

Baragwanath's story has been told in this way by some of its longest serving staff. Early on in my research process I met with two of those people: Dr Chris van den Heever and Dr Asher Dubb. Both remarkable doctors who had spent much of their working lives at Baragwanath, they were, in the hospital's vernacular, 'Bara Boeties'. ('*Boetie*' is Afrikaans for brother; Bara Boeties were those who saw themselves, and were seen by others, to exemplify the ethos and spirit of the hospital in its mythological form. A more detailed discussion of the 'Bara Boeties' is offered in Chapter 4.) Much of the existing writing on the hospital came from their pens. The enthusiasm both men had for the need to detail the history of this remarkable institution was infectious. Their generosity in sharing their knowledge and the materials they had collected marked the beginning of my quest to tell the history of Baragwanath Hospital.

I wanted to tell the story of the hospital in a more nuanced and contextualised way than the 'Bara Boeties' had done. Through the use of specific occurrences at Baragwanath and the detailed life stories of hospital administrators, doctors and nurses, I present a vibrant, vivid, nuanced and individualised account of certain aspects of the history of Baragwanath Hospital. While hospital medicine and its development form an important background to a number of chapters in this book, I do not give a full account of how hospital medicine developed at Baragwanath. I focus, rather, on certain innovations and advancements to show the broader social and political factors that contributed to their development and the importance that doctors and nurses placed on these developments when describing their experiences at Baragwanath.

This approach also enabled me to explore the institutional history of Baragwanath within the broader context of apartheid South Africa. As such, this book is not only the history of Baragwanath Hospital but also an exploration of apartheid health care and the complex and contradictory nature of institutions which functioned within the apartheid state. One of the important themes of this focus is the experiences of urban Africans, the demographic group which formed the majority of Baragwanath's patients. During the late 1980s, the renowned medical historian Roy Porter persuasively argued for a medical history written from the patients' perspectives.[19] In this book, patients' experiences have had to be accessed through sources other than their own voices. Early on in the research process, I was refused permission to interview chronic long-term patients at the hospital, which I had hoped would be a way of selecting patients. Just about every Soweto resident has had some interaction with Baragwanath and the process of gathering a representative sample would be out of the scope of my research, but it does offer rich pickings for a future study. A greater focus on patients, on a more general level, would also have shifted the focus away from the institution and its ethos which forms the basis of this study. There are, however, a few narrations from published stories, newspaper articles and patients' letters which I have used to give a glimpse into patients' experiences. It is also possible to extract a great deal of information about the experiences of patients by reading the existing source material 'against the grain'.[20] The commentary of the doctors and nurses, their official reports and other primary sources tell us much about what patients were experiencing in the hospital – even if mediated through others.

Baragwanath also does not hold inactive patient records for long, and no patient records were available for my study. During early visits to the hospital, I was told by patients that even active records are often lost. A number of patients remembered being told by nurses as far back as the 1960s to take their files home with them between visits as they would be safer. Thus, quantitative research on changing epidemiology based on patient records would be impossible. Some idea of the changing patterns of diseases presenting at the hospital can be gleaned from the journal articles and other medical publications of Baragwanath's doctors. While these articles tell us about the academic interests of doctors at Baragwanath it is unclear to what extent they actually reflect the medical needs of the population.

Works on the history of urban African health are limited. Among those that do exist, early critical works, such as Shula Marks and Neal Andersson on epidemics and social control, and Maynard W Swanson on bubonic plague, discuss the health care system for blacks as a means of controlling disease and epidemics that might affect whites.[21] These works are part of a broader historiography that addresses the relationship between the state and the provision of health care, particularly in the colonial era.[22]

Drawing on this analysis, a number of studies produced during the 1980s, as health care (especially for blacks) entered a period of crisis, analysed the broader social impact of apartheid health care. This work, much of which was done in the political economy of health mode, began to question earlier heroic models that saw increasing medical knowledge as the core factor in improving health. They saw large-scale political and economic forces as having a significant effect on health and on shaping epidemiological patterns.[23] Cedric de Beer's study of tuberculosis and of the country's health services argues that 'injustice and exploitation are as important as germs in causing disease',[24] and further suggests that 'health services are not structured as a rational response to disease. They are a state institution, and as such reflect the interests and policies of the ruling class within that state.' Marks and Anderson have shown that epidemiology is shaped by cleavages of race and class, and that the interaction of health hazards in the mining industry, migrant labour and social dislocation in the countryside, and conditions of impoverishment in towns and countryside, have created an environment where disease proliferated.[25]

For the Transvaal (now Gauteng Province) in which Baragwanath is situated, the history of urban African health care has largely focused on the mines. Soweto, despite being the province's largest and most important township, has received very little historical attention and its health care has been particularly understudied. Perhaps this was in part a result of the fact that even prior to the outbreak of violence in the mid-1970s, Soweto was a difficult place in which to conduct research, and many researchers were refused permission to work in the area. Unsurprisingly, much of the writing on the township that exists for later periods is absorbed by struggle politics, ubiquitous in Soweto from the mid-1970s, and especially on the school students' revolt of 16 June 1976. The history of Baragwanath cannot be understood without understanding the socio-political context and health status of the community the hospital served.

By dealing with the period during which apartheid was being institutionalised in the decades after 1940, through its stages of change until its tumultuous death throes in the 1980s, this book develops a fuller understanding of the shifts and, in many cases, important continuities in health care and hospital service in this understudied but important region. This is significant if we are to apprehend the intricacy of health care during apartheid. A number of studies have stressed the inequality of apartheid health generally, but very few have looked at these inequalities on an institutional level.

In South Africa there is now a burgeoning literature on the 'developmental state'. Most of this literature falls into two time-periods; the first, smaller, body of literature focuses on the pre-apartheid period and the second, more developed, body of literature focuses on the post-apartheid period. While my study is located firmly within the apartheid era falling between these two literatures, a brief exposition of their value better situates my work.

The pre-apartheid literature, formulated around the developmental state in the colonial context, has grown out of Fred Cooper's work. It has focused on institutional innovations within agricultural, welfare and economic diversification.[26] Saul Dubow, while not specifically referring to the developmental state, makes a strong argument for the state's very deliberate initiatives to create and develop scientific institutions (including medical institutions) during the early twentieth century.[27] These institutions played a major role in defining the population in ways that would shape a radicalised electorate and are indicators of the developmental state. Bill Freund is the major proponent of this literature focusing on the interwar years.[28] He argues that the hallmarks of the developmental state can be seen in the series of commissions that the Smuts government implemented which considered all aspects of the government's social and economic policy. Among the most relevant to urban African health were the Reitz Commission (1941) and the Gluckman Commission (1944). Many of these commissions led to the establishment of new institutions and parastatals which could regulate and inform overarching policies of the state beyond the work of ministries and which tended to form under the control of an elite whose key interests were the development of industrialisation and who saw the introduction of welfare policies as important only insofar as they benefited the capitalist project. Therefore these policies focused on what Freund refers to as the social engendering of a racially defined citizenry and the creation of the Bantustan system.[29] The establishment of institutions, outside of the state, which directly and indirectly shaped social welfare and economic growth within the existing racial policy, suggests that South Africa could be seen as fitting into a development state model.

The greatest part of the recent literature on the 'developmental state' and South Africa focuses specifically on the post-apartheid period. Questioning the lack of success in the post-apartheid neoliberal economy has led to a debate about the extent to which the government has, or should, adopt a democratic developmental state model. In post-apartheid South Africa, where the existence of a democratic state is fundamental to the national narrative, these discussions inevitably stress that the East Asian model can be adapted for application in a democratic milieu where the focus was on the social developmental contributions of the state. Some argue that post-apartheid South Africa is an 'intermediate' state with some of the qualities of the development state but unable to be wholly defined as such.[30] As yet little work exists on the development state during the apartheid period and this would be a worthwhile line of enquiry for scholars to pursue in future studies. As the post-apartheid body of literature develops, it would be useful to incorporate the study of a medical institution such as Baragwanath Hospital into it, to draw on Freund's argument that there were indeed some important and as yet unexplored continuities from the interwar years that survived into the apartheid era. The creation of medical schools for blacks and the creation of an urban medical centre such as Baragwanath could be seen as a form of developmentalism which fitted into South Africa's racial ideology; especially because a majority of those using Baragwanath were integral to the industrial economy. It would therefore be possible to develop this argument to interpret the provision of health care in apartheid South Africa in a way that would further nuance the apartheid meta-narrative. That, however, is not the emphasis of the current study. This empirically grounded work highlights the voices and the agency of the people involved in running and staffing the hospital. While I have drawn on Posel's argument that the apartheid state was never a hegemonic entity,[31] the primary focus is on the ways in which individual actors had the agency to work within the state to shape medical care. My study therefore focuses on the internal life of the hospital rather than the ways in which the state, externally, shaped the hospital. A micro-history of the power dynamics, work culture and the radicalised spaces of Baragwanath Hospital offers a rich case study to illustrate the contradictions which shape the internal logic of a medical institution during apartheid. In future, others may wish to build upon this work to assess how the developmental state concept could be applied to Baragwanath Hospital in a more top-down fashion than outlined here.

During the first half of the twentieth century, general hospitals such as Baragwanath became the dominant institutions in the provision of health services to urban Africans in Soweto and, indeed, in the whole of the Transvaal. This study adds to an understanding of the complex setting of general medicine. By shifting the focus away from a single disease, the focus is of necessity more general with respect to medical issues, but this also enables a discussion of competing medical needs within such a hospital. By focusing on the institutional level I highlight one of the underlying paradoxes of health service provision at Baragwanath, and more generally to black South Africans during apartheid. While my research affirms much of the general emphasis in the literature on the inadequacies of basic health care for black people, it also demonstrates that pockets of clinical excellence did exist and the hospital did offer biomedicine to black patients. Health services like those provided by Baragwanath did make a material difference in the lives of many black Sowetans and those from further afield.

In a different context, Megan Vaughan has shown that medicine, medical knowledge, biomedical practices and institutions were an integral part of the colonial project. Yet, she argues, the impact of biomedicine cannot be defined simply as an extension of the violence of colonialism.[32] This is important in the South African context as well. On the one hand, health services such as those provided at Baragwanath between 1948 and 1990 can be seen as serving the apartheid project whereby segregated African patients were often given inferior treatment and where power lay in the hands of the medical sector, creating a form of dependence. On the other hand, health services such as those provided by Baragwanath made a material difference in the lives of many black South Africans.

There were other contradictions. The hospital treated only black patients, yet segregation could never be fully carried out in its daily running where white administrators, black nurses and predominantly white doctors – of various political persuasions – worked side by side, for the nature of the work meant that strict racial segregation was impossible to enforce. There are accounts and anecdotes of racial mixing and cooperation.[33] Barriers were often broken down, at least temporarily, by the struggle to provide health care. These and other contradictions that defined the workings of this hospital within the apartheid state will be explored in the chapters that follow.

Part of the reason for the paucity of in-depth studies of Baragwanath Hospital is the lack of easily available source material, especially for the apartheid period. Although a number of records exist for the decade from 1940 to 1950, this is not the case for the period after the establishment of the independent hospital board in 1953. The major records pertaining to Baragwanath's administration were probably kept by the provincial Department of Hospital Services. I was, however, unable to locate them. They were not listed on any of the computerised accessions or national and provincial archives, and I was told that they were still in the possession of the Department. However, the Department has moved offices since 1994, and I was told that no records pertaining to the period of this study are housed at the Department of Health. One other historian had consulted some of the TPA's Department of Hospital Services records in the temporary archive depot in the mid-1990s, but my attempts to track them down there proved fruitless.

The institutional records of the hospital are also patchy. Space was at a premium and many of the older files seem to have been destroyed. Chris van den Heever remembers the administration burning records to make space for new material during the 1990s. He was able to rescue a number of documents, which now form part of his personal collection. The hospital archives have the minutes of hospital board meetings only for a period from the early 1970s onwards.

The main source of documentation on the hospital is a haphazard but intriguing collection of documents, brochures, newsletters, photographs, newspaper cuttings and other records in the storeroom of the hospital's public relations department. I was given full access to these archives and spent time in the department going through them. Here one finds copies of the hospital's internal newsletter, the 'Bara-meter', and its predecessor 'Bara-notes'. Again, limited space has shaped the collection and required successive public relations officers to select the material that would be kept. The very selection of documents remaining in the archive is revealing. While these choices obviously shaped my research, they also act as a window into what the hospital's public relations team and administration prioritised. Through their selection one can get a sense of what took place at the hospital and the image of the hospital the administration sought to portray. A telling example of this is discussed in Chapter 6.

The perceptions, motivations and experiences of doctors and nurses are central to the story told in this book – this is not, for the most part, the stuff of medical journals or official papers and nor can one rely solely on the accounts written by medical professionals, who tend to paint their engagement with the hospital in heroic terms. These works, while providing invaluable material on chronological developments and first-hand insight into aspects of the institution, leave a number of significant gaps. There is relatively little academic analysis that takes into account the broader historical and political shifts. Some of these studies address personal experiences of apartheid and hint at the ways in which apartheid affected the hospital externally, but they do not address the complex and contradictory ways in which apartheid played out *within* the hospital.

To take the reader further into the heart of the institution and to paint a vivid picture of the hospital in relation to the broader social and political context of apartheid, this book makes innovative use of alternative sources, among them the private papers of doctors and departments. In addition, because Baragwanath was often in the public eye there are a vast number of media reports spanning the period of this study.

A significant portion of this book is based on in-depth oral interviews with doctors, nurses and a limited number of other hospital professionals. These interviews were vital for accessing and analysing the distinctive disposition and individual motivations and experiences of the two professional groups who shaped the hospital.

During the apartheid era, Baragwanath employed, at any given time, approximately 500 full-time doctors and about triple that number of nurses. Many doctors who trained at Wits would, at some stage in their training, have passed through the gates of Baragwanath, especially because some of the undergraduate teaching was done there. Baragwanath's nursing college, as will be explained in Chapter 5, attracted and trained many nurses, and many other nurses came to Baragwanath to do postgraduate training and worked at the hospital for a few years to gain experience. I selected nurses and doctors from different cohorts whose collective involvement with the hospital spanned four decades. To a large extent, the doctors interviewed reflected the racial and gendered division of the medical profession. Between 1948 and 1990 the vast majority of doctors at Baragwanath were white men.

At the same time there can be little doubt that the people I interviewed were biased towards those who felt a special bond to the hospital. Those who came forward to be interviewed, or who wrote about their experiences, often saw themselves as having a stake in the hospital's history. Some had spent their working lives at Baragwanath; they were at the core of the hospital, and had shaped and responded to its ethos.

I spent a great deal of time at the hospital, often observing and engaging people in informal conversations during three periods of fieldwork, each of between three and five months, between 2003 and 2005. Although they took place a decade after the period of my study ends, these visits helped me to gain a feel for, and understanding of, the hospital as a living institution.

Organisation

Chapter 2 sets the early development of Baragwanath within the context of debates about the provision of health care for the urban African population during the late 1930s and into the 1940s. It shows how these debates were intertwined with the development of Baragwanath as an Allied military hospital and how the arguments continued with a different set of players as the military hospital was transformed into a civilian one in the same year as the National Party came to power. Here, the tensions between central, provincial and local government over the provision of urban African health care are brought to the fore.

These tensions are a constant theme in the history of Baragwanath and are picked up again in Chapter 3. The story this chapter tells is a complex one that unravels the relationships between the state, the hospital's own staff and those of Wits University. Since Baragwanth was a teaching hospital for the Wits medical school, the university added another layer of administration to Baragwanath's already complicated administrative structure. Baragwanath was, to some extent, dependent on the university for administrative support and staffing. However, merely describing the roles of these administrative bodies fails to convey their real significance on the daily functioning of the hospital. To understand this, the chapter goes on to discuss the uncertainties and ambiguities inherent in such an overlapping administrative structure which, on one level, had negative effects. Incongruously, it also had some beneficial effects. The multiple layers of administration provided the institution with a space in which to operate outside the direct purview of any of the levels of administration, and individuals could raise funds, manoeuvre professionally and influence the quality of medical care. Finally, this chapter shows the ways in which Baragwanath's status as a teaching hospital had the benefit of bringing in both equipment and highly trained staff.

Chapters 4 and 5 discuss the two professional groups at the core of the hospital, the doctors and nurses, exploring their motivations and experiences and how these changed – or in many cases remained surprisingly constant – from the first generation of medical men and women to staff the hospital in the 1940s through to 1990. These two central chapters explore one of the overriding themes of this book: that those who worked at Baragwanath saw it as a unique and special place to work and that this helped them to deal with the difficult conditions they faced. Both chapters illustrate doctors' and nurses' perceptions and both analyse why interviewees found their work at Baragwanath professionally and personally fulfilling. The chapters speak to the ways in which the identities of doctors and nurses, as 'Bara Boeties' and 'Bara nurses', were intertwined with the ethos of the hospital. At the same time, the chapters examine why nurses and doctors drew on their image of Baragwanath as being exceptional to justify their careers and to help them cope with the challenges they faced at the hospital.

Other than administrators, soldiers, police and a handful of suppliers, traders, religious and politically active people, the only white people who had a sustained relationship with the segregated township of Soweto were doctors. Interviews highlighted the contradiction that by the 1970s, the height of apartheid, when many whites sought to avoid Soweto, doctors wanted to work at Baragwanath. Many eminent doctors spent their careers there, despite the difficulties they encountered and the disparaging attitude of outsiders. These doctors spoke about the hospital in very different tones. They argued that Baragwanath offered unparalleled opportunities for professional and personal growth. Chapter 4 examines these claims by highlighting the personal histories of doctors drawn from different generations of Baragwanath's history and exploring their personalities, characters and motivations.

Unlike the doctors, most of the Baragwanath nurses during apartheid were black. When the civilian hospital opened its doors in 1948, the ward sisters were, with one exception, white. By the mid-1950s each ward was placed under the control of a registered black nurse and by the 1980s all ward sisters were black.[34] This shift suggests the desire of the increasingly segregationist state to place black patients in the care of black nurses, but it also shows the increasing importance of nursing as a profession at a time when few opportunities existed for black women. Chapter 5 turns to an in-depth discussion of Baragwanath's nurses, many of whom trained at the hospital's nurses' college. They also had varying reasons for taking up nursing. For some, altruistic motives such as helping the sick, and a religious calling to the profession, were important. Other important motivations were specific to the context of apartheid South Africa: the important status that nursing brought to black women and the fact that nursing education was funded. In other ways too, nursing at Baragwanath was the story of nursing during the apartheid era. Nurses at Baragwanath were part of what Shula Marks has called a 'divided sisterhood'; [35] part of a broader sisterhood of nurses who shared a profession – yet they were black women in apartheid South Africa and never fully accepted into the white-dominated nursing hierarchy. Against this background, the nurses in this study developed their own identity not only as black nurses but specifically as Baragwanath nurses.

Many of these issues are highlighted by examining three specific events that took place at Baragwanath during the period of my study: a threatened strike in 1949; a one-day strike against the introduction of passbooks for women, beginning with nurses, in 1958; and a major strike by almost 2 000 student nurses and daily-paid workers in 1985. These events are used as examples of moments of crisis which, as Helen Sweet and Anne Digby have discussed with regard to nurses' strikes at mission hospitals in South Africa, highlight deep divisions of race, gender, hierarchy and specific patterns of power.[36] The incidents show that the changing nature of apartheid and nursing legislation, and broader political shifts, all had significant effects on the issues that sparked nurses to take action, the nature of their action and the responses to their action. These actions are also significant in South African apartheid history because they are examples of women mobilising women at a time when public politics was dominated by men. At the same time, the strikes reveal the complex identity of the nurses, both as part of the 'divided sisterhood' and as 'Bara nurses'. By letting the voices of individual nurses come to the fore we are able to develop a more nuanced understanding of the way nurses defined their role and place in the history of the hospital.

Chapter 6 uses two case studies, and the state response to them, to demonstrate the central contradiction in Baragwanath's service delivery, and an important ambiguity in apartheid medicine more generally. Firstly, the story of the 'successful' separation of the conjoined Mathibela twins at Baragwanath in 1988 shows how Baragwanath's image was communicated locally and internationally. The operation became an icon of the sophisticated and advanced medical specialisation that was available at Baragwanath to the country's black population. At the same time, the simmering issue of persistent overcrowding at the hospital was thrust into the public eye by a letter of protest signed by 101 Baragwanath doctors. The original letter, which derided the deplorable conditions at the hospital, was printed in the *South African Medical Journal* in September 1987. The circumstances surrounding the writing of the letter, and the subsequent fallout, will be used as a case study to highlight the other side of Baragwanath. The chapter shows that while attempts were being made to publicise excellence in black health care, little was actually being done at the hospital to ease congestion or improve the horrendous conditions. These two cases are thus two sides of the same coin and represent the contradiction at the heart of apartheid medicine – and the central theme of the book. These cases show the very real material benefits of western biomedicine that the state provided to the African population but the difficulties that a majority of the population had in accessing these benefits.

The phoenix of Baragwanath as a military hospital was born among arguments about urban African health care. It lived its life among the young men battered by war and the women of South Africa, Canada and the United Kingdom who tended them. It died surrounded by disputes very similar to those which were the chorus of its birth. Out of these ashes was born a phoenix whose life and death was filled with the complex contradictions and continuities of delivering health care in apartheid South Africa. That phoenix has died with the changes in health legislation in the early 1990s. The phoenix of the post-apartheid era is still in its infancy.

Endnotes

1   'Intake Night – Baragwanath Hospital' by Mbuyiseni Oswald Mtshali, courtesy of the poet, from *Sounds of a Cowhide Drum – Imisindo Yesigubhu*

Sesikhumba Senkomo. Johannesburg: Jacana, 2012. (First published by Renoster Books, 1971).

2   'Baragwanath Hospital' by Oupa Thanda Mthimkulu in *Staffrider* 1 (1978).

3   K Huddle and A Dubb (eds) (1994) *Baragwanath Hospital, 50 Years: A Medical Miscellany*. Johannesburg: Department of Medicine, Baragwanath Hospital, p. v.

4   Bara PR Archives, History File, L Spies 'The History and Establishment of Baragwanath Hospital: A Comprehensive Overview of the Establishment of the Hospital and its History up to 1980' (unpublished paper, c. 1980), p. 1.

5   Chris van den Heever (24 January 2003) VdH Papers, B Lawson 'The Development of the Maternity Ward at Baragwanath' (unpublished paper, June 1980).

6   I Frack 'Guest Editorial: Baragwanath Hospital, Decennial Anniversary'. *Medical Proceedings*, 4:10 (17 May 1958), p. 250.

7   D Posel (1997) *The Making of Apartheid, 1948–1961: Conflict and Compromise*. Oxford: Clarendon Press.

8   See, for example, A Jeeves 'The Role of Health Assistants and Health Educators in South Africa's Experiments with Primary Health Care in the 1930s and 1940s' (unpublished paper, presented at American African Studies Association Annual Meeting, Washington, DC, 17–20 November 2005) and earlier published work including S Marks (1997) 'South Africa's Early Experiment in Social Medicine, Its Pioneers and Politics'. *American Journal of Public Health* 87, pp. 452–59.

9   HC Van Rensburg and D Hamson (1995) 'History of Health Policy'. In D Harrison *South African Health Review 1995*, p. 59.

10   M Foucault (1973) *The Birth of the Clinic*. London: Pantheon.

11   L Granshaw (1997) 'The Hospital'. In WF Bynum and R Porter (1997) *Companion Encyclopaedia of the History of Medicine*. London: Routledge.

12   C Rosenberg (1987) *The Care of Strangers: The Rise of America's Hospital System*. New York: Basic Books, pp. 5–6.

13   R Porter 'The Gift Relation: Philanthropy and Provincial Hospitals in Eighteenth-Century England'. In Granshaw and Porter op. cit., pp. 149–78.

14   Rosenberg op. cit. Studies such as PV Pickstone (1985) *Medicine and Industrial Society: A History of Hospital Development in Manchester and its Region, 1752–1946*. Manchester: Manchester University Press seek to place the history of the hospital within the broader context of urban history.

15 GB Risse (1999) *Mending Bodies, Saving Souls: A History of Hospitals.* Oxford: Oxford University Press.

16 JTH Connor (1990) 'Review Essay: Hospital History in Canada and the United States'. *Canadian Bulletin of Medical History* 7, pp. 93–104.

17 EH Burrows (1958) *A History of Medicine in South Africa up to the End of the Nineteenth Century.* Cape Town: Balkema; PW Laidler and M Gelfand (1971) *South Africa: Its Medical History, 1652–1898.* Cape Town: Struik.

18 A Digby, H Phillip, H Deacon and K Tomson (2008) *At the Heart of Healing in Cape Town: Groote Schuur Hospital, 1938–2008.* Johannesburg: Jacana.

19 Cf. R Porter (1985) 'The Patient's View: Doing Medical History from Below'. *Theory and Society*, 14, pp. 167–74; R Porter and D Porter (1989) *Patient's Progress: Doctors and Doctoring in Eighteenth-Century England.* Cambridge: Cambridge University Press.

20 AL Stoler (2002) *Carnal Knowledge and Imperial Power: Race and the Intimate in Colonial Rule.* Berkeley: University of California Press, p. 83.

21 S Marks and N Andersson (1984) 'Epidemics and Social Control in Twentieth Century South Africa'. *The Society for the Social History of Medicine Bulletin* 34, pp. 32–4, and MW Swanson (1977) 'The Sanitation Syndrome: Bubonic Plague and Urban Native Policy in the Cape Colony'. *Journal of African History* 18: pp. 387–410.

22 For a general overview see S Marks (1997) 'What is Colonial about Colonial Medicine? And What Has Happened to Imperial Health?' *Social History of Medicine* 10: pp. 205–19.

23 Key studies in this mode include: S Marks and N Andersson (1987) 'Issues in the Political Economy of Health in Southern Africa'. *Journal of Southern African Studies* 13: pp. 177–86; R Packard (1990) *White Plague, Black Labour: Tuberculosis and the Political Economy of Health and Disease in South Africa.* Scottsville: University of Natal Press; K Jochelson (2001) *The Colour of Disease: Syphilis and Racism in South Africa, 1880–1950.* Basingstoke: Palgrave. For a similar approach elsewhere in Africa, see M Turshen (1984) *The Political Ecology of Disease in Tanzania.* New Brunswick: Rutgers University Press.

24 C de Beer (1986) *The South African Disease: Apartheid Health and Health Services.* London: Africa World Press, p. 78.

25 Marks and Andersson (1987) op. cit., p. 117.

26   Cf. Fred Cooper, *Decolonisation and African Society: The Labour Question in French and British Africa.* Cambridge: Cambridge University Press, (1996).

27   This argument is advanced most notably in S Dubow (2006) *A Commonwealth of Knowledge: Science, Sensibility, and White South Africa, 1820–2000.* Oxford: Oxford University Press.

28   Bill Freund *A Ghost from the Past: The South African Developmental State of the 1940s,* (cf 34), (unpublished paper, presented at the University of KwaZulu-Natal).

29   W Freund (2007) 'South Africa as Developmental State'. *Africanus: Journal of Development Studies,* 37:2, pp. 191–198.

30   R Southall (2006) 'Can South Africa be a Developmental State?'. In S Buhlungu et al. (eds) *State of the Nation: South Africa 2005–2006.* Cape Town: HSRC Press.

31   Posel (1997) op. cit.

32   M Vaughan (1991) *Curing Their Ills: Colonial Power and African Illness.* Palo Alto: Stanford University Press.

33   Desmond Pantanowitz (15 July 2004); Yehuda Kaplan (1 March 2004); Harriet Gwebu (16 August 2003); Annah Ntshangase (19 August 2004).

34   Bara PR Archives, History File, L Spies 'The History and Establishment of Baragwanath Hospital: A Comprehensive Overview of the Establishment of the Hospital and its History up to 1980' (unpublished paper, c. 1980), p. 4.

35   S Marks (1994) *Divided Sisterhood: Race, Class and Gender in the South African Nursing Profession.* London: St Martin's Press.

36   H Sweet and A Digby (2005) 'Race, Identity and the Nursing Profession in South Africa, c. 1850–1958'. In B Mortimer and S McCann (eds) *New Directions in the History of Nursing in International Perspective.* London: Routledge, pp. 109–124.

CHAPTER 2

From Allied Military Hospital to Urban African Hospital

What was new and exciting about this convoy [of ambulances and buses] on May 1st 1948 was that it was conveying non-European patients to their own hospital on its opening day, and for them this was a move from grossly overcrowded conditions at the Non-European Hospital in Johannesburg to a place of quietness and light and, above all, a place where each patient had a bed to sleep on and space to move about freely.[1]

The 'place of quietness and light' was Baragwanath Hospital. Ironically, within a few years of its opening the hospital became so overcrowded that few patients had a bed to themselves and there was very little 'space to move about freely'. Yet the early excitement about the opening of Baragwanath as a civilian hospital for black patients should be seen in the wider context. From the early debates about the establishment of Baragwanath as an Allied military hospital in the early 1940s to its subsequent acquisition by the Transvaal Provincial Administration (TPA), Baragwanath's history was deeply intertwined with arguments about the provision of urban African health care. The story of the birth and death of Baragwanath's first phoenix and its place within the context of urban African health care is important in itself. But the early years also saw the foundation of a specific Baragwanath ethos, for the staff in the early years were those who practised medicine in difficult under-resourced situations – military or civil – and thrived. They developed innovative solutions that they were proud of, and they often stressed the mutual support and assistance created by working in such conditions.

Soweto and its health services, pre-1948

The area today known as Soweto was given its name in 1963 – a composite, coined from the first two letters of each of the words South Western Township.[2] The first of the sub-townships or suburbs was formed in 1905 when the Johannesburg City Council used an outbreak of bubonic plague as a stimulus to clear a Johannesburg slum where Africans and Indians had been living. Over one thousand Africans were moved to Klipspruit. At the same time it became illegal for Africans to live in the city unless they were living in compounds at one of the mines, or working as live-in domestic workers in homes in the white suburbs. The move met with opposition from both workers and employers, as Klipspruit was about eight miles from the centre of town and transport was limited, unreliable and expensive. In the face of mounting opposition, the Johannesburg City Council granted employers permission to develop private compounds on their land for their employees. Policing those who lived in these compounds proved difficult and they tended to become overcrowded living spaces for the ever-increasing number of Africans flocking to the Witwatersrand (now known as Gauteng, 'Place of gold' in Sesotho).

Conditions in Klipspruit were no better than they had been in the slums and although health concerns were given as a justification for the move, little was done by the municipality or health department to provide health care or to improve conditions. Tenants who rented land or huts from the municipality had sewerage and water charges built into their rent, but the many people living in overcrowded backyard rooms had access to few lavatories or taps and no water-borne sewerage – and the site was also surrounded on three sides by a municipal sewerage farm.[3] This, together with inadequate infrastructure and services, led to extremely high incidences of infectious disease and a high infant mortality rate which saw thousands of babies die each year, a rate that was higher than in Johannesburg as a whole.

The slums terrified white Johannesburg. They were seen as dens of iniquity, filled with illicitly brewed liquor, prostitution, disease and racial mixing. The 'sanitation syndrome'[4] referred to the exploitation of diseases by the authorities for the implementation of segregationist social policies when the metaphorical equation of urban Africans with disease and contamination became a significant justification for residential racial segregation.

It is unsurprising that in the first two decades of the twentieth century the provision of health care, slum clearance and ideas of urban segregation were deeply intertwined. This is not to suggest a direct link between the outbreak of disease and the passing of segregatory legislation, but it points to the complex dynamics behind the politicisation of disease and the broader socio-economic framework surrounding illness. Around the country, increasing urbanisation, the development of slums, outbreaks of bubonic plague (1901), smallpox (1912) and Spanish influenza (1918), as well as increased cases of venereal disease and tuberculosis, focused the attention of authorities and ordinary people alike on issues of health and disease.[5]

The high death toll of the 1918 Spanish influenza, especially among the African population, led to a renewed urgency in urban reform. One way in which this played out was through the passing of the 1919 Public Health Act, which had as much to do with segregationist concerns as with health. It was used to regulate European residential conditions and urban planning and also provided many municipalities with another way of regulating African urbanisation and enforcing segregation under the guise of health concerns.

The Act was the first attempt to coordinate the country's health care on a national level under a fully-fledged department of health, but it did little to consolidate health service delivery. It placed a minority of hospitals, mostly tuberculosis, leprosy and psychiatric hospitals, under the control of the central government. The Transvaal Provincial Administration (TPA) retained responsibility for the establishment, maintenance and management of general hospitals as originally directed in the South African Act of 1909. Responsibility for preventing the spread of disease, and for hospitals dealing with infectious diseases, fell to local authorities, although the division of responsibility in these multiple layers of administration was far from clear.

During this period, the Johannesburg City Council was making some attempts, albeit motivated by racial paternalism, to provide services for those already living under their charge – but the provision of curative health fell to the provincial administration and the main centre at which urban Africans could access curative care (outside of the mines) was some distance away from major African settlements, at the Non-European Hospital. In reality the Non-European Hospital was a ward of the Johannesburg General Hospital, but by 1929, four years after its establishment, the Non-European Hospital had only 206 beds.[6] Because of this shortage, the council derived authority from the Native (Urban Areas) Act to provide curative services in Pimville. These services, begun in 1927, employed a part-time medical officer to oversee them.[7] At this point medical services were already in short supply, and the situation got worse with migration to the cities and accelerated urban slum clearance.

In the 1930s the context in which slum clearance took place changed. The Great Depression from 1929 saw a quickening of both white and African migration to the towns. This movement was intensified by the effects of the devastating drought that gripped South Africa in 1932–3. Simultaneously, many landowners were keen to dispense with their white tenants or *bywoners* during the interwar years, so that they could extend commercial agriculture. The result was an increasing number of poor Afrikaner farmers moving into cities in search of a better life; many found themselves living in the urban slums, which exacerbated fears of racial mixing.

It was not only these push factors which increased migration to the Witwatersrand, or 'Rand'. New employment opportunities were opened up by the industrial growth which followed South Africa's abandoning of the gold standard late in 1932. The rising price of gold also led to a rise in revenue for the Union government – revenue they were happy to spend on furthering segregation and creating new townships.

Against this background, the African township of Orlando, adjacent to Klipspruit/Pimville, was established by the Johannesburg City Council. This marked the beginning of modern Soweto. Much attention was paid to the planning of the township. Houses were to suit 'a better-class native, the new Bantu who has a sense of beauty and proportion'.[8] In reality the accommodation was inadequate, far from workplaces and lacking almost all community amenities. One of the few amenities provided in the township, however, was a small municipal clinic which opened in 1932. The following year a small cottage hospital, a gift bequeathed by Mrs Corlett, wife of DF Corlett who was the mayor of Johannesburg from 1931 to 1932, opened with two wards – six beds in each – and a small operating theatre. Once built, the hospital was equipped and run by the Native Affairs Department.[9] In the years prior to the establishment of Baragwanath these were the only government-run institutions providing hospital-based medicine to patients closer to their homes than the Non-European Hospital, twelve miles away.

There were, of course, alternative nongovernmental medical practitioners who also offered health-related services on the Rand. These included African diviners (*isangoma*), herbalists (*inyanga*) and those who healed within religious frameworks. Many indigenous healers from different ethnic backgrounds flocked to the Rand, where the heterogeneous waged population offered a ready market.[10] A number of independent doctors – often of Jewish or Indian ancestry – also saw African patients,[11] although they could not practise in the urban townships under the regulations of the Group Areas Act of 1923, so access to their services was limited and fairly expensive.[12] There were also a limited number of African doctors who, having qualified abroad, returned to South Africa, and worked on the Rand.[13] All these forms of health care were, however, limited by the apartheid state, either though witchcraft legislation, which sought to control indigenous healing, or through the policies of segregation and oppression.

Health care developments in the Soweto area before World War Two

The population of Soweto has proven notoriously difficult to determine, much of it migrant and mobile and living in unofficial squatter camps. Although legally required to register births, deaths and marriages, many avoided doing so, in part because they might not have had the correct documentation to be living in Soweto and would wish to avoid being recorded in any official sense. However, some population estimates for the regions which would become Soweto have been made through a few censuses or by researchers working in the area. In 1935, Orlando had 3 000 houses which were home to 18 000 people.[14] In the wake of increasing slum clearance this area grew dramatically in the following decade. During the 1940s Orlando's 5 000 properties housed 35 000 people. The 1946 census put the population of Orlando at 57 461 and Klipspruit/Pimville at 16 616. By the middle of the following decade there were over 200 000 people in Orlando and its adjoining townships. Two decades later it was estimated that the Soweto population was between 1 and 1.5 million. The 1980 census put the figure at 860 000 but it is generally accepted that this underestimates a population of which, by the 1980s, at least a third was illegal.[15] Some of the Baragwanath doctors suggested that by the 1980s the population of Soweto might have been as high as 2.5 million.

The growth of these areas also led to an increasing demand for medical and other services. For the white populations in the surrounding areas the growing townships caused anxiety and fear about the spread of disease, and they demanded controlled segregation and health care. For the African population, demands focused on medical care and housing.

During World War Two, the need for accommodation in the vicinity that was to become Soweto increased exponentially while the number of houses built remained almost static. Overcrowding was becoming especially acute in Orlando, where thousands lived as sub-tenants in small, four-roomed houses – and there were thousands of homeless people elsewhere on the Rand. Out of this housing shortage grew the squatter movement, a key leader of which was James Mpanza, founder of the Sofasonke movement in Orlando. Under Mpanza's charismatic leadership, sub-tenants and homeless migrants settled on a vacant piece of land in Orlando West. Mpanza became a surrogate for the Johannesburg City Council, allocating sites and setting up a rudimentary administration.[16] The movement and its subsequent waves played a large part in compelling the Council to develop alternative accommodation in the area which became Soweto. Much of this accommodation was temporary and of a poor standard. In some areas, such as the emergency camp of Moroka, residents had to build their own shacks and only limited services were provided by the municipality. One service provided in Moroka in 1947 was a clinic located in a large tent.

The Johannesburg City Council provided a part-time medical practitioner to visit each of the four major Rand townships (Western and Eastern Native Townships, Pimville and Orlando) three times a week at set hours. There were also two resident nurses/midwives in each township. During the 1940s, a further clinic was established in Jabavu, which would later become part of Soweto, and in the townships of Shantytown and Noordgesig. These services, however, only went part of the way towards filling the demand for biomedical services.[17]

In the pre-war years, the national Department of Public Health was led by individuals who had a progressive social welfare approach and who seriously considered a number of social reforms,[18] but this short window of progressive leadership had limited effects on the health care of urban Africans. Hospital services were insufficient and health care delivery uncoordinated. The overriding focus, for all arms of government, remained segregation rather than health care improvements.

The start of World War Two sparked a major political crisis that brought about the dissolution of the government and the resignation of the prime minister, Barry Hertzog, who did not favour entering the war. In September 1939 Jan Smuts became prime minister and led South Africa into the war on the side of the Allies. The war stimulated the already diversifying economy and further increased the demand for manufacturing; to meet the consequent demand for labour, pass laws were temporarily relaxed. African migration to Johannesburg gathered momentum. According to the census of 1936, the African population of Johannesburg reached approximately 200 000; a decade later the figure had risen to almost 300 000 and the 1951 census recorded the black population of Johannesburg at 500 000. By the mid-1950s, the Witwatersrand had come to house about 1.6 million black people, making it home to the largest urban black population in South Africa – and probably in sub-Saharan Africa. The state faced major problems in providing services for this rapidly growing population.

Throughout the 1940s there was an increasing awareness, at least among some officials, of the desperate need for hospital care for the urban African population. A series of reports, letters and press articles put pressure on the national and provincial authorities to make improvements to the health care facilities. In 1942, for example, the Smit Committee reported the high incidence of ill-health among urban Africans and the inadequacy of preventative and curative care,[19] recommending that 'there should be an expansion of hospital, dispensary and district nursing and midwifery services for urban natives'. In 1948 the Fagan Commission pointed out the inevitability of African urbanisation and the need to provide services. It was amid these debates that discussions about the establishment of Baragwanath as a military hospital became intertwined with the concurrent deliberations about urban African health care.

The war years and the debates about the establishment of Baragwanath as a military hospital

In 1939, Britain, and indeed the entire British Empire, was suffering from backlogs in the provision of health care for military personnel. As hostilities escalated in the early 1940s, the need for additional hospitals and convalescent facilities became urgent. There were already base hospitals in Egypt at Alexandria and Cairo, but Italian colonies lay between the Allied troops in the north and south. There was still a need for additional hospital accommodation for Allied troops.[20] Despite its distance from the front, South Africa was considered a suitable location. The country had a long history of providing hospital services for the Imperial forces – during the First World

War the wounded were housed at hospitals in Natal and at the Cape in Maitland and Wynberg. At the outbreak of the Second World War, Union troops were hospitalised near Pretoria, at Voortrekkerhoogte, which had about 400 beds. An additional twenty-five beds were available at the military hospital at Wynberg and there were 120 beds at a hospital taken over from Premier Mines. Small camp hospitals were also set up around the country, and hospitals such as the Johannesburg General Hospital, Addington Hospital and Groote Schuur set aside beds for military use. But these turned out to be not enough, and soon after the beginning of the war additional hospital accommodation was already being considered.

The British War Office asked the Union Government to provide a 2 400-bed hospital and a convalescent depot. Sir Edward Thornton, South Africa's secretary of public health from 1932 to 1938, and director general of medical services, advised that one hospital and depot should be built in Port Elizabeth and another near Johannesburg.[21] Thornton had a career-long involvement with military medical services. During the First World War he had been responsible for coordinating the provision of military hospitals for South African troops and had also served as superintendent of a military hospital in the Cape. While Port Elizabeth (which was on the coast and easy to reach by ship) was considered, only one hospital – in Johannesburg – was ultimately built. Durban, rather than Port Elizabeth, became the main port for hospital ships. Johannesburg and Durban were linked along the main railway line and it was considered best to keep hospitals along this line. Johannesburg also had a well-developed health infrastructure with a university medical facility that had been in operation since 1922. It offered a climate ideal for the recovery of those suffering from diseases such as tuberculosis, and was free of tropical diseases like malaria. It had nurses' training colleges and rehabilitation facilities. Baragwanath began life as a military hospital in Johannesburg.

It is unlikely, however, that the decision of where to place the hospital could have been made without an awareness of the desperate need to provide health care for the many Africans now living around Johannesburg. By the 1930s there had been a gradual and grudging acceptance of the presence of a permanent urban African population, partly as a result of the manufacturing industries' support for a settled labour force.

There were only 400 general hospital beds at the Non-European Hospital and a small number of additional beds at three private hospitals. Two of these, the Bridgman Memorial Hospital in Johannesburg and the Princess

Alice Hospital in Sophiatown, were maternity hospitals,[22] while the third was Nokuphila, a small twenty-bed hospital run by the Seventh Day Adventists, in Western Native Township.[23] The Johannesburg Hospital Board made numerous appeals to the TPA for two large new hospitals, one at Orlando for African patients and another at Coronationville to serve all sectors of the 'non-European' population, but the TPA rejected these requests. In 1941, while debates about construction of a military hospital in the Soweto region continued, the TPA once again refused the Hospital Board's request for the creation of additional hospitals to serve urban Africans. They argued that a military hospital would be built in the region and could be converted into a civilian hospital at the end of the war, and that a further 150 beds for the chronic sick would be provided at Rietfontein. At the same time, they suggested that there were insufficient funds to undertake the establishment of a hospital at Coronationville.[24] This exchange is important because it shows the TPA's conviction that the military hospital would be built with the dual purpose of serving soldiers during the war and becoming a civilian hospital for urban Africans afterwards.

The Johannesburg Municipality and the Department of Public Works examined a number of sites, all of which were near the Baragwanath aerodrome, which had been Johannesburg's leading air force facility since 1919. It also happened to be in the vicinity of the developing townships of Orlando and Pimville. The Department of Public Works considered three sites; sites A and B were on council-owned land, while the third site was not. Site B was situated between the two railway lines in the vicinity of Nancefield Station and between the Pimville and Orlando 'locations' (townships) and would be an excellent place for an African hospital after the war. That, however, was the site's only advantage. Not only was it too small for the proposed 1 600-bed hospital, but it was also waterlogged owing to the distribution of sewerage effluent over the area – hardly the ideal location for a hospital. At the same time, the clay-rich subsoil made an unsuitable foundation for buildings. Site A, on the other side of the railway line from site B, appeared to be just as waterlogged. The sites could not be joined to solve the size problem, and both seemed unusable.[25]

The third site, on high ground nearer to the entrance of Orlando, was accessible, and had relatively dry soil that would hold the foundations of a large building. However, the council did not own this land on Diepkloof farm. Crown Mines Ltd held the surface rights to the land but they held no mining title. Negotiations were immediately entered into with the mining company, which sold a 100 acre portion of ground to the Union government, which in turn granted it to the British government, rent-free for the duration of the war.[26] By November 1941, as things continued to look bleak for the Allies, there was an urgent need to construct the hospital as quickly as possible and construction started under the auspices of the Red Cross.[27] The Johannesburg municipality contributed water, electrical and sewerage services, and agreed to construct roads and paths within the site at a minimal profit.[28]

The style in which the hospital was built bears the marks of its dual purpose. Many military hospitals in South Africa at the time consisted either of hutments in existing barracks or under canvas, but Baragwanath was planned by the Department of Public Works to be a permanent structure, which greatly increased the costs. The British, who funded the building works, agreed to the extra cost on condition that it would be repaid when the South African civilian authorities took over the hospital.[29] Its layout was military in design. It was built in the Pavilion architectural style that had been popular in Britain from the 1850s until the late 1930s.[30] The buildings were designed for convalescent patients and were barrack-like, single-storey pavilions. The principal advantage of Pavilion architecture was the ease with which units can be renovated without disturbing neighbouring wards, and the speed with which further units can be added. This design allowed the hospital to be divided into geographic areas serving particular medical disciplines. There were, however, several disadvantages. They made for a disjointed, sprawling hospital where wards, theatres and administration buildings were scattered and often linked only by open-air pathways.

By May 1942, less than six months after construction began, the Imperial Military Hospital Baragwanath was ready to admit its first patients. The entire facility was complete within eighteen months. The speed of construction was achieved by the employment of several contractors simultaneously. At the opening of the hospital in September 1942, Field-Marshall Jan Smuts stressed the importance of the envisaged role of the hospital when he stated:

When the war is over there will remain a great need to look after the health of the native population gathered on the Rand. Then Baragwanath might turn out to be one of the most useful institutions in the country. We had planned along these lines and I wish Baragwanath a most useful career, not only in this war but in the long period thereafter.[31]

This speech reflects the rhetoric of the time about the provision of hospitals for the urban African population but the central government proved reluctant to pay for the conversion of the hospital after the war.

British and South African military doctors staffed Baragwanath. White women, local and foreign, made up the nursing staff. The early history of nursing in South Africa was closely linked to the United Kingdom through the work of religious sisterhoods at both missionary and non-missionary hospitals. During the South African War (1899–1902), and in the decades that followed, a number of volunteers, only some of whom were qualified nurses, flocked to South Africa. These were women from Britain, Europe, Australia and Canada. When World War II broke out many of them, as well as their South African compatriots, volunteered to serve on the fronts.[32]

Increasingly short of nurses to staff the newly established military hospitals, the Union government approached the Canadian Government in mid-1941 to request permission to second three hundred Canadian nurses to serve in South Africa during the war.[33] Ottawa agreed and the first group of eighty Canadian graduate nurses arrived in Cape Town aboard the ship *SS Kawsar* in December 1941. They then headed by train to Durban and on to various military hospitals, including Baragwanath. (Gladys J Sharpe, the matron of the Toronto Military Hospital, who was to serve as the first matron of the Baragwanath Military Hospital, was aboard the *El Nil*, the second ship bringing Canadian nurses to South Africa in February 1942.) A third group of nurses, most of whom served at Baragwanath, arrived aboard a convoy of ships in July 1942.[34] These nurses brought with them an image of nursing in the mould of Florence Nightingale, in their secular volunteerism and in how they perceived and presented the profession of nursing. It was an image of nursing that had already been introduced to South Africa in the nineteenth century by an English Anglican nun, Sister Henrietta Stockdale, and one that continued to be felt at Baragwanath during the apartheid era.

The South African contingent who staffed Baragwanath as a military hospital were trained nurses belonging to the South African Nursing Corps, and lay volunteers. One of the approximately 200 volunteers who served at Baragwanath during the war remembers how 'there were different groups of us, we were trained at different sites. I was trained by St John's Ambulance at the Cullinan Mine Hospital. We spent six weeks there ... I was sent to Bara in May 1942'.[35] These volunteers assisted the nurses with daily chores, such as making beds, cleaning and dressing patients, and preparing food. Despite the presence of volunteers, the wards were becoming understaffed even before the conversion of the hospital into its civilian form. One ex-patient remembered that 'those noble women had volunteered their services up to certain dates and time was up for many of them and it was "civvy street" for them now. They just slipped out of our lives unobtrusively.'[36] At the same time, many of the Canadian nurses who had filled the posts in the early years of the war left South Africa.[37]

Baragwanath's shift to a civilian hospital, 1946–8

Early in 1946, negotiations began for the transfer of Baragwanath to the Transvaal Provincial Administration. On one issue there seemed to be consensus: there was an urgent need for a civilian hospital to serve the ever-expanding African population around Johannesburg. The actual process by which Baragwanath became the hospital serving that community was more complicated. The original agreement was between the British and the South African governments; however, the handover actually involved not only the transfer of the hospital to the national government but also its further transfer to the TPA, under which fell the administration of hospitals for black patients. The debate rested on questions of the suitability of the hospital for use as a general hospital – and who should pay for its transfer. These questions were part of a broader protracted struggle between the national and the provincial authorities regarding jurisdiction and health care.

A second, slightly less contentious, issue was what to do with the large number of imperial troops still in the hospital. Both governments agreed to retain Baragwanath as a military hospital until the end of 1947 but no patients would be admitted after October 1946. The South African Department of Health also decided that the remaining patients would be transferred to Britain when a military ship became available and when conditions in Britain were considered acceptable. If this proved impossible, they would be moved to other South African hospitals, such as Voortrekkerhoogte, the Union Military Hospital at Roberts Heights. Those who returned to England were promised continued support from the Red Cross.[38] At the same time the secretary for health, George Gale, attempted to find places for individual patients in existing provincial TB hospitals.[39] While Baragwanath had originally been equipped to deal with medical and surgical cases, as the war progressed most patients admitted were suffering from TB and the hospital, in a good location as Johannesburg's warm dry winters were ideal for recuperating TB patients, developed special facilities and personnel for the medical and surgical treatment of tuberculosis.[40] By 1944, the hospital was operating solely as a tuberculosis convalescent home for Allied soldiers.

The decision to delay the transfer of the hospital by a year meant that Baragwanath was still a British military hospital when the royal family came to South Africa on an official visit in April 1947. The king, queen and princesses Elizabeth and Margaret visited on their 'free' day, 5 April 1947. They met and decorated senior military and medical staff, and visited patients in the wards. A number of the patients were also decorated with medals such as the Distinguished Service Cross.[41] The royal visit temporarily shifted the focus from the debate over the transfer of the hospital, but the lull was short-lived.

Almost a year after the negotiations for the handover of Baragwanath begun, it emerged that the papers detailing previous discussions were incomplete and it was still unclear what ministerial consultations had taken place.[42] These doubts meant that earlier debates about the suitability of the hospital briefly returned. It was clear that the provincial administration wanted to gain control of the hospital but did not want to bear the considerable conversion costs. Assuming that the national government would carry a large portion of conversion costs, the TPA argued that the hospital was suitable for use as a civilian hospital. The TPA also reminded the government that they had been involved in the planning stages on the basis that Baragwanath would become a provincially-administered civilian hospital after the war.

To add weight to their argument that the conversion costs should be carried by the national government, the TPA claimed that Baragwanath would have national importance, as a civilian hospital, in the training of black hospital personnel. George Gale, the national secretary of health, suspected that the provincial administration was using this argument to prepare the ground for a free transfer of the hospital on the basis that it was serving a national function, and contended that other hospitals in the vicinity could provide these facilities and that the main obstacle to the training of black doctors was the lack of posts for black nurses. Black nurses would have to staff wards in hospitals where black doctors were being trained to avoid a situation where a black houseman would give orders to a white nurse – a situation wholly unacceptable in South Africa.[43] The argument over the national function of the hospital proved fruitless and the sides were no closer to an agreement about who should bear the conversion costs.

By February 1946, an estimated £400 000 was owed to the British government for construction expenses. The TPA acknowledged this but refused to also acknowledge that this was the worth of the hospital to the administration, arguing that because the hospital was built as a war emergency hospital designed for speed of completion and not for economy of function, it was not built in a way that was beneficial to them. They claimed that the lack of a casualty or outpatient department, an outdated heating system and the fact that the staff housing consisted of merely a military camp, would be costly to deal with – and they suggested that the valuation should be halved, to £200 000, or that the Union government should assist with the costs.[44]

The continued dispute created a major dilemma for the Union government which was still determined to use Baragwanath to deal with the lack of hospital services for urban Africans. As such there was pressure to turn the hospital over to the TPA and have it operating as soon as possible, even if this meant meeting the TPA's demands. But there was no precedent for them to follow. The Treasury feared that the assistance of the Union government in a TPA purchase of Baragwanath would result in other provinces, and indeed other hospitals in the Transvaal, demanding a *quid pro quo* in the form of grants to convert or build their own hospitals.[45] Towards the end of 1947, the TPA finally agreed to pay £400 000 for the hospital primarily because they, like the Union government, saw Baragwanath as a solution to the provision of urban African hospital services. It was, after all, the TPA that bore ultimate responsibility for hospital care.[46]

The TPA had gained authority for all hospitals in the province in 1946 though an amendment to the 1919 Public Health Act which not only dropped the word 'public' from the title of the national department but also placed executive authority for health care in the hands of the Department of Health while decentralising other functions. Hospitals remained firmly in the control of the provincial authorities who dealt with their establishment, staffing, hospital policy and equipment. Thus, in 1948, under the auspices of the TPA, a civilian 'phoenix' arose. The hospital opened with 480 beds. Administratively, Baragwanath fell within the ambit of the Johannesburg Hospital Complex, and the Johannesburg Hospital Board was responsible for its operation.

A dedicated team was set up to oversee the conversion of the facilities at Baragwanath. JD Allen, who had recently applied for the post of deputy superintendent of the Johannesburg Hospital, was appointed as superintendent. He had eleven years of experience in general practice, had held senior administrative posts in military service and had experience as superintendent of Germiston hospital. The rest of the team consisted of Jane McLarty who had, for the previous eight years, been matron of the Non-European section of the Johannesburg Hospital, and GR Kempff, who became the hospital secretary. This team not only oversaw the physical transformations of the hospital but also had an influence on its founding ethos. Both McLarty and Allen were deeply invested in training African health care professionals and both strove to deliver the best health care it was possible to deliver to Africans during the apartheid era.

The first thing this group of early administrators had to contend with was a new set of debates. Although the arguments about the suitability of Baragwanath as a civilian hospital seemed to have been settled on a political level, they still had to be considered on a medical level. The level of modification to convert the hospital varied substantially between departments. Some aspects needed little modification – in a letter to Dr W Waks, the acting medical superintendent of Johannesburg, the professor of surgery, William Underwood, suggested that: 'the operating theatre is suitable in every way and will be quite adequate for the work. It is taken that the theatre equipment be included in the "take over", this is important.'[47] In other areas the hospital was not well suited to its proposed purpose. The site was not quite as accessible as originally thought. There had been talk, within the health department, about the possibility of extending the railway and placing a station at the entrance to Orlando, which would be nearer to the hospital than the station at Nancefield, nearly four miles away,[48] but this never came about. Even getting to the front gates was a challenge. Patients often had to run the gauntlet of heavy traffic that passed the hospital entrance at all hours.

Much of the conversion work was completed in conjunction with Wits, which was committed to using Baragwanath to train both black and white students. In May 1947, the Wits registrar, I Glyn Thomas, outlined to Waks, the acting superintendent of the Johannesburg Hospital, what the university required: this included residential accommodation for 120 black students and ten white students. The Hospital Board, with provincial administration agreement, allocated a site on the southern boundary (some distance from the wards) to the university to erect a hostel. The hostel, common rooms and lavatories were all segregated.

The phoenix of the civilian hospital took its first tentative flight in December 1947. By this time, overcrowding at the Non-European Hospital had become acute and hospital authorities decided that the preliminary opening of a few wards at Baragwanath would be a simple way of relieving the pressure. Just over one hundred patients and temporary staff were moved. In January 1948, the first component of civilian medical staff were appointed: twenty full-time senior staff and an additional five part-time senior staff as well as fifteen intermediate and thirty-one junior staff. The nursing body was made up of forty-five trained white nurses, sixty-three trained black nurses and 282 student nurses, all of whom were black.[49]

They had between January and April 1948 to prepare for the 'great move' of patients. The move, which began on 29 April, was planned with military precision. The first patients to be moved were those suffering from infectious diseases and those who were seriously ill. After that, the transfer of patients moved into full swing. Superintendent Allen called the days on which the move was planned 'D-Day, D-Day+1, and D-Day +5'. Each patient had a serial number tied to a buttonhole with a tag containing information about the patient and to what ward they would be admitted at Baragwanath. D-Day was Saturday 1 May, when 250 patients were to be moved. The first two wards cleared were then used as the evacuation centre. On the following day, another 250 patients were moved. On Thursday 6 May the final 100 patients were moved. Within five days, between 700 and 800 patients, together with staff, were moved from 'the grossly overcrowded conditions at the Johannesburg Hospital to the more spacious and newly-reconditioned wards at Baragwanath Hospital'.[50]

Staffing the civilian hospital: The first generation and their legacy

The first groups of doctors to work at Baragwanath after it was converted to a civilian hospital were a mix of ex-army and civilian doctors from South Africa and from the United Kingdom (many of the latter were specially recruited British civilian doctors who played an important role in academic medical education; this group will be discussed in more detail in Chapter 3). The

South African staff component was made up of army doctors who remained at the hospital, a number of doctors who moved with the patients from the Non-European wing of the Johannesburg Hospital, and a group of doctors who moved from other hospitals. The staff also included the first groups of medical interns to be sent to Baragwanath when an additional year of practical experience and training became compulsory in South Africa in 1948.

This combination of local and foreign doctors set in place a foundation and ethos that became the basis for a shared account of Baragwanath's specific and unique identity, an identity developed and communicated through the ranks of the staff and to the outside world. It was not always easy to discern and extract the motives of doctors on the basis of their own explanations, comments and writings, and there are of course always different shades of motivation, yet many of the beliefs instilled at the hospital by these early doctors remained remarkably continuous, at least in the minds and words of a core group of doctors in the decades that followed. These doctors, and to some extent the early senior nurses who joined them, became legendary in their own right. Later generations referred to the pioneers – or the mythologised versions of them – to explain what they believed to be the special and unique character of the hospital and to link them to a broader fellowship of 'Bara' staff.

Among the South Africans recruited to Baragwanath from other hospitals was John Donald Allen. He was transferred from Germiston Hospital, where he had been the superintendent, to oversee the conversion of Baragwanath and to become its first superintendent. From a missionary family, Allen was born and educated in South Africa and served in the South African Medical Corps during the Second World War. He played an important role not only in the physical conversion of the hospital but also in instilling a positive tone among the staff. He appears to have been well-liked and respected. When he died, four clerks, writing on behalf of black hospital staff, emphasised the integrity and leadership of the man they called *Lethola Ramosa* (the quiet, merciful and most kind-hearted one), and point out that to Allen, 'the lowest member of his staff was worthy of consideration irrespective of colour or creed'.[51] While obituaries are standardised in their style and format and are most often praising and triumphant, the image of Allen presented complements other descriptions. The hospital administration also seemed to have recognised his commitment to all levels of staff when they instituted prizes for the best nurse and non-nursing staff member (the JD Allen Incentive Prizes) in his honour.

His role in shaping the ethos of the hospital was also acknowledged by his colleagues. In a letter to the Baragwanath Hospital Medical Committee, the head of the Department of Surgery, Libero Fatti, suggested that it would be:

> fitting that [Allen's] good work in promoting the good spirit and efficient activity of Baragwanath Hospital in its first-decade should be commemorated. A suitable memorial would be to name the new operating theatres whose existence we owe to him 'the JD Allen Theatres' and that a suitable tablet be put up in the main entrance of the Block.[52]

The new DJ Allen theatres were opened in November 1957. In many senses the block serves to commemorate the man as well as the distinctive approach he represented. Allen was a leader with a positive attitude who respected all levels of staff and all races. More than a decade later, the mayor of Johannesburg, Patrick Lewis, in his address on the occasion of Baragwanath's twenty-first birthday also commented on Allen's legacy saying that 'all who knew him pay tribute to his ability, his leadership, his inspiration in creating the atmosphere which, from the start made Bara a happy hospital – a hospital with which people wanted to be associated'.[53]

For many of the young students, interns and registrars who arrived at the hospital in 1948, Baragwanath was an exciting place to work in. It was a hospital that served a clear need. It was also a new development, which meant that doctors working there would have the opportunity to shape innovative clinical practices. At the same time, the combination of local and foreign doctors drawn from both military and civilian backgrounds promised a distinctive learning experience. There were many reasons for optimism in the early years.

This first generation of students, including Asher Dubb, Thomas Bothwell, and DJ (known as Sonny) du Plessis, remained connected with Baragwanath for much of their working lives. Dubb became professor of Medicine at Baragwanath, serving there until he retired in the early 1990s; Bothwell became dean of the Faculty of Medicine at Wits after serving many years at Baragwanath; Du Plessis was professor of Surgery at Baragwanath from 1958 to 1977 and then became vice-chancellor at Wits. Baragwanath attracted staff drawn from different backgrounds: the three doctors were from Jewish, English and Afrikaner families respectively. They valued the opportunities the hospital offered, and as teachers they passed their enthusiasm for and dedication to the hospital to the next generation.[54]

Not everyone, however, was as positive about the new hospital. In fact, there was reluctance on the part of some South African doctors to be associated with it. Reflecting on what he had been told about the early years of the hospital, Van den Heever explained that it was widely perceived that when Baragwanath opened 'the guys at Johannesburg [Hospital] did not want to come and work here, it is too far'. One gets the sense that 'too far' implied physical distance but also the idea that as a black hospital it would be on the periphery of medicine in South Africa. This was one reason for the shortage of local doctors to staff the wards and to fulfill Baragwanath's purpose as a teaching hospital during the late 1940s. Another reason, as discussed in the previous chapter, was the reluctance to train and hire black doctors.

The TPA focused on recruiting local white doctors who were, in the early years, almost exclusively trained at Wits. This changed little throughout the apartheid era but what was unique to this period was the recruiting of mainly British staff to academic positions. Beginning in 1948, one of Baragwanath's largest departments, the Department of Medicine, was led by three British physicians: James Gilroy, Vernon Wilson and Alexander Duncan Gillanders, a Scotsman who had trained at the Royal Infirmary, Edinburgh. The biographies of these men show South Africa's place in the broader process of empire mobility. In the colonies, medical appointments were used as a way to consolidate power.

Gilroy was born in South Africa, during the Siege of Ladysmith (1899–1900) according to the mythology surrounding him, but was brought up in the UK. In August 1947, Gilroy wrote to Mills, the superintendent of Johannesburg Hospital, to apply for a physician post at Baragwanath or Coronation Hospitals. It seemed that he was keen to work in South Africa and specifically at one of the hospitals serving black patients. Gilroy had experience with and an interest in tropical medicine after having worked in North Africa, the Sudan, British Guyana and in the Amazon. He felt that a hospital like Baragwanath would suit his professional development.[55]

Vernon Wilson's biography is not entirely clear. Popular anecdotes about him suggest that he was sent to South Africa from India during the war with a serious lung condition and was admitted to Baragwanath.[56] I have, however, found no evidence that this was so. Rather, it seems that Wilson, already a qualified physician, was involved with work on treating pulmonary tuberculosis while stationed in South Africa. It also seems that his medical discharge from the army, in 1944, was due to diabetes mellitus and not a lung complaint.[57] Gilroy's and Wilson's links to South Africa were often emphasised by other doctors and members of the hospital administration as an explanation for their commitment to the country and their special links to Baragwanath.

The first head of the Department of Surgery was Libero Fatti, born in South Africa in 1901. He attended school at St John's College and then studied medicine at University College London, specialising in cardio-thoracic surgery before returning to South Africa to take up the post at Baragwanath in 1948. He was joined by G Reginald Crawshaw, one of the recruits from the United Kingdom.[58] South African born Samuel Skapinker, a Wits graduate who had served in the East African, Middle Eastern and Italian campaigns during the war before specialising in surgery at the University of Edinburgh, became the third head of the surgical unit at Baragwanath. Godfrey Phillips Charlewood, another South African, who would eventually head obstetrics and gynaecology, was also in this group of doctors.

This early staff did some remarkable research, completing theses as well as publishing medical books and articles in prestigious journals. They made an important contribution to Baragwanath's image as a site of world-class research. Three major pieces of research by staff members appeared in the hospital's first year.[59] In 1949, four articles appeared in international journals. In 1950 there were fifteen publications from Baragwanath – eight of these in international journals. This early research focused on pulmonary diseases, tropical diseases and stab wounds, all of which were prominent epidemiological features of the urban African population of the Witwatersrand. Unsurprisingly, then, these were themes that became a staple of Baragwanath research.

On arrival at Baragwanath, Wilson had been told that patterns of disease in black patients differed strikingly from that of whites and that black patients were unable to withstand serious injury or major surgery.[60] These perceptions were based on broader racist assumptions which had a long trajectory in South Africa. Saul Dubow has shown that the interest in comparative physiology dates back to the early twentieth century: scientists, palaeontologists and other experts began a detailed examination of fossil remains as they began to solidify their work on human origins and racial typology.[61] These studies were augmented by a set of research imperatives which sought to dissect and study the entire African body. The appointment of Australian anatomist and anthropologist Raymond Dart to the newly-established department of anatomy at Wits brought this agenda into the university. In 1937, Dart expanded on this research agenda that called for 'an army, equal to that which has laboured in Europe over the last 400 years since Vesalius, [to be] organised in Africa to collect information about the Bantu similar to that which has been garnered over these centuries concerning Europeans'.[62] Dart, who discovered the hominid fossil known as the 'Taung child', sought to explore the possible evolutionary connection between early hominids and modern Africans. As Philip Tobias, one-time student and eventual successor of Dart pointed out, in the decade that followed, '[e]very day, instances of variation in some anatomical feature or other are brought to light in work on the Bantu on the operating table, in the post-mortem and in the dissecting-hall'.[63]

Against this background Wilson found that '[t]hese discouraging administrative and clinical observations attracted rather than discouraged interest in our "opening batsmen" who were drawn from people with conviction and untiring enthusiasm'.[64] While a full review of the work of these doctors remains to be done, a preliminary overview suggests that instead of allowing these suppositions to influence the type of medicine they practised, many of the early doctors set out on clinical investigations that did not assume inherent racial difference. They sought, rather, to understand the diseases they saw around them, and found that assumptions about the incidence of disease amongst Africans were based more on a lack of clinical data than any accurate understanding of disease patterns. Wilson found that the research at Baragwanath was 'referable to both European and non-European problems'.[65] Similarly, Kleinot pointed out that '[n]o one will deny that in the study of Bantu pathology and disease processes generally lies the key to many problems affecting the whole range of medicine in its direct application'.[66] This research was taking place against the background of broader changes in the way the state and medical authorities had come to view Africans. Ideas of inherent difference and unsuitability to urban life were giving way to a gradual acceptance of an urban African population and an acknowledgement of the social and environmental causes of disease.

One of the major research projects undertaken in this vein was on cancer. The key researcher was John Higginson, an Irish immigrant to South Africa with a degree in pathology from Glasgow. Higginson was appointed to the staff of the pathology laboratory of the South African Institute of Medical Research (SAIMR) at Baragwanath in 1949. Over the next decade, drawing much of his research data on black patients from Baragwanath, Higginson played a key role in the institute's study of the incidence of cancers in different ethnic groups in South Africa. The study's ultimate object was to determine the environmental factors that accounted for the racially defined differences in the incidence and epidemiology of cancer.[67]

Another example of early work at Baragwanath that sought to investigate the degree to which Africans were significantly medically different from whites was that of obstetrician and gynaecologist Godfrey Charlewood. In the introduction to his 1956 study *Bantu Gynaecology*, his colleague OS Heyns suggests that

> [l]ess than twenty years ago the Bantu were an exotic growth to the gynaecologist. Now this branch of the human race has been received in orthodox gynaecological circles, and its womanhood forms for the observer an entity ... The first question that arises about the material is the racial one, and it would be of value to establish whether this people offers anything unusual in character and behaviour and what is its origin'.[68]

The book is made up of a number of examples of diseases and disorders that are either more common in black women (such as tuberculosis of the female genital tract and gynaecological schistosomiasis) or, like genital prolaps, are significantly less common in black women than white. In each case Charlewood argues that there is no proof of a correlation between racial difference and epidemiology, and that environmental factors seem more significant. This type of research had, as both Didier Fassin and Alexander Butchart have pointed out, a profound influence on the shaping of racial segregation. Both authors draw on a Foucaudian analysis to show the ways in which such racialised research shapes social identity both through a process of 'othering' and through the ways in which it is used to justify state power.[69] Seen though this lens, the work these early doctors were doing was both scientific and (consciously or subconsciously) political. Despite their varied reseach and the diverse political positions they took, these doctors played a joint role in shaping the clinical medicine practised at the hospital and also the ways in which health and health care became contested ground within the apartheid state. At the same time they were part of the creation of a cultural environment that became the foundation of the mythology that later defined the hospital. Many of them spent decades working at Baragwanath. They were committed, and demanded commitment from those they taught. They set the tenor of what was expected of a 'Bara doctor' in years to come. The story of Baragwanath's later generations of doctors will be picked up again in Chapter 4, which will show the continuities in the way doctors viewed their identities, the hospital and their roles within it even as they faced new challenges and the practice of medicine developed in significant ways. The professional reasons for working at Baragwanath which were stressed by these early doctors, remained, perhaps counter-intuitively, remarkably consistent in doctors' own narratives across the generations.

Endnotes

1   'Baragwanath Hospital Twenty-First Birthday', *Rand Daily Mail*, 26 March 1969.

2   I have, throughout this book, used the term 'Soweto' to describe the area, even for periods prior to its naming, for ease of discussion.

3   WJP Carr (1990) *Soweto: Its Creation, Life and Decline*. Johannesburg: South African Institute of Race Relations, pp. 11–2.

4   Swanson op. cit., pp. 387–410.

5   On plague, see for example Swanson op. cit. On Spanish influenza, see H Phillips (1990) *Black October: The Influence of the Spanish Influenza Epidemic of 1918 on South Africa*. Pretoria: Government Printer. On venereal diseases, see Jochelson op. cit. On tuberculosis see Packard op. cit.

6   SAB, JHM 89, 583/49 'Johannesburg Hospital: Growth and Development during the Period 1929–1949' Report by KF Mills (no date), pp. 1–2.

7   'Medical Services: Native Townships – History of the Service'. Minutes of the Mayor, Johannesburg City Council, 4 November 1938–2 November 1939, p. 221.

8   *Umteteli wa Bantu*, 30 January 1932, cited in P Bonner and L Segal (1998) *Soweto: A History*. Cape Town: Maskew Miller Longman, p. 16; and P Lewis (1969) *'City Within a City': The Creation of Soweto*. Johannesburg: Wits University Press, p. 5.

9   Johannesburg City Council, Minutes of the 564th Meeting, 28 March 1933, paragraph 262. By 1941 the hospital provided mainly maternal and child care.

Anthropological and sociological works giving examples of plural health-seeking practices during this period in urban areas include E Hellmann (1948) *Rooiyard: A Sociological Study of an Urban Slumyard*. Oxford: Oxford University Press, p. 138; and L Longmore (1959) *The Dispossessed: A Study of the Sex-life of Bantu Women in Urban Areas in and around Johannesburg*. London: Cape, pp. 231–2, 245–7.

11 TD Wilson (1984) 'Health Services within Soweto', Second Carnegie Inquiry into Poverty and Development in Southern Africa, Paper No. 170, 13–19 April, p. 4.

12 KA Shapiro (1987) 'Doctors or Medical Aids: The Debate over the Training of Black Medical Personnel for the Rural Black Population in South Africa in the 1920s and 1930s'. *Journal of Southern African Studies* 13, pp. 234–55.

13 For a general overview on the early training of black doctors and particularly on Silas Modira Molema see A Digby (2005) 'Early Black Doctors in South Africa'. *Journal of African History* 46:3: 4A, pp. 427–54. On AB Xuma see ZK Matthews 'A Tribute to Late Dr AB Xuma' *Imvo Zabantsundu*, 10 February 1962; AB Xuma 'Native Medical Practitioners' *The Leech*, 5 (November 1933), pp. 12–5; and on James Moroka see LR Olivier and JR Kriel 'A Job Well Done – a Short History of Dr James Moroka' *South African Medical Journal*, 54:8 (19 August 1978), pp. 331–2; Digby op. cit.; and on Dilizantaba Mji see WHP, A2675, Folder 23, Karis/Gerhart Collection, Transcript of interview with D Mji by G Gerhart, p. 1. Diliza Mji talks briefly about the medical career of his father, Dilizantaba.

14 E Hellman (1971) *Soweto: Johannesburg's African City*. Johannesburg: South African Institute of Race Relations, p. 4.

15 P Morris (1981) 'Soweto: A Brief History'. *The Black Sash* 24:2, August: 7–13, p. 8.

16 AW Stadler (1979) 'Birds in the Cornfields: African Squatter Movements in Johannesburg, 1944–1947'. *Journal of Southern African Studies* 6, pp. 94–9; Bonner and Segal op. cit., p. 19; K French (1983) 'James Mpanza and the Sofasonke Party in the Development of Local Politics in Soweto'. University of the Witwatersrand, MA thesis.

17 Annual Report of the Medical Officer of Health, City of Johannesburg, year ending 30 June 1949, pp. 5, 12.

18 A Jeeves (2001) 'Public Health in the Era of South Africa's Syphilis Epidemic of the 1930s and 1940s'. *South African Historical Journal* 45, p. 81. See also Marks (1997) op. cit., pp. 452–9.

19   Report of the Inter-Departmental Committee on the Social Health and Economic Conditions of Urban Natives, Smit Committee, G.P. 57272-1942-3 (Pretoria, 1942), Chapter V, paragraphs 86–133.

20   HJ Martin and N Orpen (1979) *South Africa at War, Military and Industrial Organization and Operations in Connection with the Conduct of the War, 1939–1945.* Cape Town: Purnell, p. 96.

21   Op. cit., p. 2 079; Van den Heever C (1993) 'Baragwanath Hospital – the Beginning'. *Adler Museum Bulletin* 19:1, March, p. 10.

22   SAB, GES 1205, 23/19, 'Johannesburg Hospital, Memorandum on the need for Additional Hospital Accommodation for Natives', 9 October 1941.

23   Minutes of the Mayor, Johannesburg City Council, 6 November 1936– 4 November 1937, p. 252.

24   SAB, JHM 116, 615/49-51 'Non-European Hospital Services: Johannesburg' Provincial Secretary H Pentz to Superintendent of Johannesburg Hospital, K Mills, 12 September 1941.

25   SAB, PWD 1064, 8/2547, Holdgate (District Representative, Public Works) to Lt Col Norburn 'Proposed Hospital in the Orlando area of Johannesburg', 6 February 1941, p. 2.

26   SAB, GES 1440, 466/19, Letter from director general of medical services to the secretary of defence 'Site for Imperial Hospital: Johannesburg', 24 April 1941.

27   SAB, PWD 1064, 13/2547 Red Cross – St John National Coordinating Committee to secretary of defence, 24 June 1946; SAB, PWD 1064, 13/2547, Letter from PB Smuts, secretary for defence to secretary for public works, 18 April 1947.

28   SAB, PWD 1064, 8/2547 Holdgate op. cit., p. 3.

29   SAB, PWD 1064, 13/2547 Letter from PB Smuts, secretary for defence to secretary for public works, 18 April 1947; SAB, PWD 1064, 13/2547 Red Cross – St John National Coordinating Committee to secretary of defence, 24 June 1946.

30   J Taylor (1997) *The Architect and the Pavilion Hospital: Dialogue and Design Creativity in England 1859–1914.* London: Leicester University Press, p. vii.

31   Speech by J Smuts at the opening of the hospital 23 September 1942 reported in the *Star,* 24 September 1942. King George VI had bestowed the rank of field-marshal on Smuts in 1941.

32   Marks (1994) op. cit., pp. 46–7 and 127.

33 WR Feasby (1953) *Official History of the Canadian Medical Services, 1939–1945: Organization and Campaigns.* Ottawa: Cloutier, p. 325.

34 CSM Girard (1983) 'Canadian Nurses in the South African Military Nursing Service: Some Reminiscences Forty Years Later'. *Military History Journal* 6:1, June, pp. 6–10.

35 Telephone interview with Mrs G Broekman, 13 July 2004.

36 B Cousins (1990) 'Heroes in White'. *Adler Museum Bulletin* 16:2, July, pp. 2–6.

37 Marks (1994) suggests that most of the Canadian nurses left after just a year. Feasby (1953) however implies that many of the Canadian nurses renewed their contracts for at least a second year: Feasby op. cit., p. 325; Nicholson (1975) believes that at least two-thirds renewed their contracts; Nicholson op. cit., p. 176.

38 SAB, JHM 121, 625/48(1), memorandum from medical superintendent at Baragwanath to heads of departments – Johannesburg Hospital, 'Transfer of Patients for Non-European Hospital to Baragwanath', 14 April 1948; SAB, JHM 121, 625/48(1); letter from the secretary of the General Hospital of Johannesburg to the Red Cross, 29 January 1948.

39 SAB, GES 1440, 466/19, letter to the minister of health from the secretary of health, Dr GW Gale 'Transfer of Baragwanath Hospital to the Transvaal Province', 6 February 1947.

40 Bara PR Archives, W Philips 'Baragwanath Military History' (unpublished paper, 6 April 1992), p. 2; W Philips 'Baragwanath Military History', *Adler Museum Bulletin* 19:3 (December 1993); 'Lady Duncan Opens Hospital Centre: New Occupational Therapy Workshops at Baragwanath' *The Star*, 22 May 1943.

41 SAB, GES 1440, 466/19, Boucher, 'Royal Visit, South Africa' (no date), p. 55; Van den Heever (1993) op. cit., p. 12.

42 See, for example, SAB, GES 1440, 466/19, letter from director general of medical services to the secretary of defence, 'Site for Imperial Hospital: Johannesburg', 24 April 1941. SAB, GES 1440, 466/19; memorandum to the secretary of health (GW Gale) from the under-secretary (H Pentz), 'Baragwanath Military Hospital' 13 February 1947, pp. 1–5.

43 SAB, GES 1440, 466/19, letter to the minister of health from the secretary of health, Dr GW Gale, 'Transfer of Baragwanath Hospital to the Transvaal Province', 6 February 1947.

44   SAB, GES 1598, 6/623/11, 'Baragwanath Military Hospital', provincial administrator to secretary of public health, 6 August 1947; SAB, GES 1598, 6/623/11, secretary to the Treasury from provincial secretary, 'Baragwanath and Tara Hospitals', 8 April 1948.

45   SAB, GES 1440, 466/19, memorandum to the secretary of health (GW Gale) from the under-secretary (H Pentz), 'Baragwanath Military Hospital' 13 February 1947, pp. 3–4; SAB, GES 1440, 466/19; memorandum from the secretary for health (GW Gale), to the minister of health (H Gluckman), 'Transfer of Baragwanath Hospital to the Transvaal Province', 27 February 1947.

46   SAB, GES 1598, 6/623/11, secretary of public works to secretary to the Treasury, 'Baragwanath Military Hospital', 21 October 1947.

47   SAB, JHM 118, 625/46-47, WE Underwood to W Waks, 9 May 1947.

48   SAB, GES 1440, 466/19, memorandum to the secretary of health (GW Gale) from the under-secretary (H Pentz), 'Baragwanath Military Hospital' 13 February 1947, p. 5.

49   SAB, JHM 121, 625/48(1), Johannesburg Hospital, 'Press Statement: Baragwanath Hospital', 27 April 1948.

50   SAB, JHM 121, 625/48(1), JD Allen (superintendent Baragwanath), to heads of departments – Johannesburg Hospital, Transfer of Patients from Non-European Hospital to Baragwanath, 14 April 1948.

51   RA Caldwell (1957) 'In Memoriam'. *South African Medical Journal* 31, p. 182 and I Frack (1958b) 'In Memoriam: John Donald Allen OBE 1900–1957'. *Medical Proceedings* 4:10, May, p. 253.

52   VdH Papers, Minutes Thirty-Fifth meeting of the Baragwanath Hospital Medical Committee, February 1957, p. 3.

53   VdH Papers, 'Speech of the Mayor, Councillor Patrick Lewis, on the Occasion of the 21st Birthday Celebrations of Baragwanath Hospital', May 1969.

54   TM Bothwell (1993) 'Some Aspects of Research at Baragwanath Hospital in its Early Years'. *Adler Museum Bulletin* 19:2, July, p. 16; A Dubb (1988) 'Baragwanath Hospital 1948–1972: The Department of Medicine: The First 25 Years'. *Adler Museum Bulletin* 24:1/2, July, p. 3.

55   SAB, JHM 121, 625/48(8), Correspondence between Dr JC Gilroy and KF Mills, Superintendent of Johannesburg Hospital, August–November 1947.

56 Bothwell op.cit., p. 16; VdH Papers, 'Speech of the Mayor, Councillor Patrick Lewis, on the Occasion of the 21st Birthday Celebrations of Baragwanath Hospital', May 1969. The same story is told by Hunt about a Dr Watson, who bears remarkable similarities to Wilson: JA Hunt (2002) *White Witchdoctor: A Surgeon's Life in Apartheid South Africa*. Dallas: Durban House, p. 59.

57 SAB, JHM 121, 625/48(8), Application from VH Wilson to KF Mills, superintendent of Johannesburg Hospital, 20 September 1947.

58 HH Lawson (1994) 'The Department of Surgery, Baragwanath Hospital – the Early Days', *South African Journal of Surgery* 32:1, March, p. 36; A Dubb (nd) 'The Chris Hani Baragwanath Hospital: A Brief History', unpublished paper.

59 A Altmann (1948) Malignant Malnutrition, Kwashiorkor. *Clinical Proceedings* 7, p. 2; Charlewood GP (1948) 'Cardiac Arrest: Modified Technique of Cardiac Massage'. *British Medical Journal* 2, December, p. 1 023; L Hirsowits (1948) 'Typhoid Fever in the Bantu' (University of the Witwatersrand MD thesis).

60 VH Wilson (1958) 'Ten Years' Medical Experience at Baragwanath Non-European Hospital'. *Medical Proceedings* 4:10, May, p. 251.

61 Dubow op. cit, pp. 208–9.

62 R Dart (1937) 'Racial Origins'. In I Schapera (ed.) *The Bantu Speaking Tribes of South Africa*. London: George Routledge & Sons, p. 31.

63 P Tobias (1947) 'Studies in Bantu Anatomy: Introduction', *The Leech*, 17:1:17 cited in A Butchart (1997) 'The "Bantu Clinic": A Genealogy of the African Patient as Object and Effect of South African Clinical Medicine, 1930–1990'. *Culture, Medicine and Psychiatry* 21, p. 414

64 Wilson (1958) op. cit., p. 251.

65 SAB, GES 3012, 8, Vernon Wilson, senior physician, 'Memorandum upon the Facilities for Medical Research at Baragwanath Hospital, Johannesburg', March 1955, p. 2.

66 SAB, GES 3012, 8, S Kleinot, senior surgeon, 'Baragwanath Hospital, Research' 15 March 1955. A similar point is also made in I Segal, ARP Walker and D Parekh (1994) 'Gastroenterology. In K Huddle and A Dubb (eds) *Baragwanath Hospital, 50 Years: A Medical Miscellany*. Johannesburg: Department of Medicine, Baragwanath Hospital, p. 17.

67 M Malan (1988) *In Quest of Health: The South African Institute for Medical Research, 1912–1973*. Johannesburg: Lowry Publishers, 1988), pp. 7, 29, 74, 197–8.

68   GP Charlewood (1956) *Bantu Gynaecology*. Johannesburg: Photo Pub. Co. of SA, pp. 1–2.

69   D Fassin (2007) *When Bodies Remember: Experiences and Politics of AIDS in South Africa*. Berkeley: University of California Press (see specifically p. 144) and A Butchart (1998) *The Anatomy of Power: European Constructions of the African Body*. London: Zed (specifically Chapter 9).

CHAPTER 3

Apartheid and Administration
The Hospital, Provincial Administration and the University of the Witwatersrand

The apartheid structures and policies had direct and indirect adverse effects on the health status of the majority of black South Africans. They also had a negative effect on the institutions offering care. Yet it is important not to see the negative structural impositions as monolithic. Since Union in 1910, South Africa's health services have been characterised by a multiplicity of health care authorities and systems rather than any single unified system. Baragwanath Hospital found itself answering to two, sometimes competing, masters in the post-1948 period. The hospital functioned under the auspices of the Transvaal Provincial Administration (TPA) but it was also one of the main teaching hospitals of the University of the Witwatersrand. The needs, approaches and politics of each of these groups fundamentally shaped health care for the African population of Soweto and the hospital.

In a 1976 article, J de Beer, secretary for health, stated that: 'looking at the health service in South Africa today we find a structure which is almost bewildering in its complexity and diversity and certainly much maligned for its fragmentation'.[1] This was nothing new in the mid-1970s. As early as 1928, the annual report of the Department of Public Health had called for better coordination of the different branches of the health infrastructure. Two decades later, evidence given to the National Health Services Commission during the early 1940s often referred to the country's disordered structure of health care services. For example, the evidence of Sir Edward Thornton, director general of medical services, described the health care infrastructure as an 'unworkable tangle of conflicting interests and jurisdictions'.

Throughout the apartheid period the South African health care system was divided according to race and geographic area. There were significant inequalities between black and white, rural and urban, and primary and tertiary health care. In addition to the public sector, there was a private health care sector catering mostly to the white population.

Similarly, the structure of hospital services – especially those serving the urban African population – suffered from what was, at best, a continual predicament of numerous overlaps and, at worst, chaos. Attempts by the central health authorities to establish coordinating councils failed. The National Department of Health, the Native Affairs Department, the Transvaal Provincial Administration and local councils continued to offer some degree of health service, sometimes complementary and sometimes leading to lengthy debates in Parliament about divided responsibilities. Baragwanath, as a teaching hospital, and Wits, were mutually dependent for administration and staffing. The university was represented on the hospital board and, in a reciprocal arrangement, the superintendent of the hospital and deputy superintendent sat on the board of the university's Faculty of Medicine. All this fragmentation had both disadvantages and benefits for Baragwanath. Many in Baragwanath were able to use it to their advantage by operating outside the direct focus of any of the levels of control or by navigating the system to their own (and sometimes their patients') benefit. These opportunities, however, did little to improve the provision of health care to the majority of urban Africans. The hospital and its resources could not keep pace with their rapidly increasing numbers, and the benefits of fragmentation did not deal with the sources of disease rooted in the appalling social and economic conditions of apartheid.

Urban African health care under apartheid

South Africa's political scene changed when DF Malan's National Party won the 1948 election and began cementing the policy of apartheid. This did not mean that all services to Africans were suspended, but some, including health services, changed shape. While the need for a healthy workforce and fears for whites' health were driving forces behind health service provisions, the National Party's views of African urbanisation are also important factors in understanding how health care services were provided to the urban African population.

Upon attaining power, the National Party argued against the existence of a permanently urbanised African population and saw very little need to fund or provide an urban African hospital. The central government maintained that, in keeping with the Public Health Act of 1919, hospital services were not its concern and that the provincial administrations had autonomy over the provision and control of these services.[2] The TPA was faced, alone, with the reality of providing hospital care for Soweto. From its health budget, the TPA funded and equipped Baragwanath Hospital and took part in appointing its doctors. Although senior doctors in public hospitals which were also teaching hospitals often held joint posts with the university, all doctors in the public service were subject to provincial terms of employment – the university paid only a small percentage of their salaries. The hospital superintendent was accountable only to the provincial authorities. The provincial authorities were, as will be shown in Chapter 6, aware of what was going on within the hospital and reacted harshly to any criticism. Finally, it was the responsibility of the local council to maintain non-medical services such as water, electricity and laundry, and to provide ambulance services.

The day-to-day operation of the hospital was under the superintendent and matron who originally reported to the Johannesburg Hospital Board. It is significant that Baragwanath, as a black hospital, was placed under the stewardship of another hospital despite the fact that the core administrative staff had a great deal of experience running various hospitals in the Transvaal. Only in 1953 did the hospital become an independent unit with its own hospital board. It included the superintendent, hospital secretary, chief matron, representatives of the hospital's doctors and four to eight white Johannesburgers with an interest in health care. The new board had direct representation to the Hospital Services Department of the TPA. In April 1954, the Baragwanath Hospital Medical Committee was inaugurated. This committee included doctors from different departments as well as the superintendent, whom they advised on medical matters. Two members of the medical committee also served on the hospital board. Baragwanath's own staff had a far greater say in hospital operations than they had had in previous years.

The hospital did, however, remain squarely within the control of the TPA, which maintained jurisdiction over public hospitals as outlined in the 1919 Public Health Act. The passage of the Public Health Amendment Act of 1952 withdrew some of the local authorities' rights and, in an attempt at unification, placed certain aspects of health services such as salaries and the running of outpatient clinics totally under the purview of the provincial administrations.

The funding of salaries, supplies, buildings and maintenance at Baragwanath also remained the duty of the TPA.

The 1960s was a particularly bleak time for urban Africans as apartheid laws became more entrenched. During this decade, the focus on Bantustans and rural 'development' took precedence over urban development and received a large share of government funding.[3] The building of houses in Soweto, which had increased after the war and with the squatter movements, slowed to a trickle. Little was done, on either a national or local level, to improve conditions at Baragwanath. Yet evidence suggests that there were some advantages for the hospital during this time – especially for Baragwanath's black staff. More weight was being given to the recommendations of the black advisory boards such as the Orlando Advisory Board. In health circles, Harriet Shezi became the first African matron in the Transvaal in 1958.[4] Baragwanath was also increasingly handing authority to African staff.[5] By this time all ward nursing was by black nurses and during the early 1960s the first three black matrons, I Maponyane, H Ndlovu and V Mkhwanazi, were appointed at Baragwanath.[6] The number of black matrons rose quickly but it was not until 1985 that the first black nurse, Jane Ramaboa, become the first black chief matron (officially her designation was senior nursing services manager) at Baragwanath.[7] Also during this period, Dr WM Matsie, the first black medical houseman at Baragwanath, became the first black doctor to teach white medical students doing a rotation at the hospital.

The focus on curative care at this time also benefited the hospital and resulted in significant expansion. In the ten years between 1958 and 1968, the number of beds increased from 1 600 to 2 347.[8] During 1957 the hospital treated an estimated 500 000 patients, including those admitted and those treated in outpatient departments. About 1200 patients passed through casualty and outpatient services every day with this number increasing to over 2000 on weekends.[9] The daily number of in-patients during the early 1960s averaged around 2 000, and the hospital was admitting between 70 000 and 75 000 patients into the wards every year. By the end of the decade the hospital was admitting about 77 000 patients and tending about 740 000 outpatient and casualty cases per year. In 1968, Baragwanath performed 25 471 surgical operations and provided care during 24 627 births.[10]

The staff complement also went up during this period. In the late 1950s there were about 230 qualified black nurses and 160 full-time doctors. By the early 1960s the hospital was employing 408 qualified nurses and 216 doctors.[11]

The complement of full-time doctors increased to 225 in 1967 and by the following year the hospital was employing 571 trained nurses, while a further 668 student nurses and 200 student midwives were registered at the hospital.[12] The unit cost per patient day also rose; however, expenditure per patient day at Baragwanath remained significantly lower than at the Johannesburg General Hospital, the comparable hospital for white patients in Johannesburg. For example, in 1963 the unit cost per patient day at Baragwanath was R3,14 while at the Johannesburg General it was R7,84. A decade later the cost at Baragwanath was R7,73 while at the Johannesburg General it had become R23,77.[13] While the inequality in levels of funding between black and white hospitals remained and while Baragwanath was underfunded for its size and patient load, its budget did increase throughout the period under discussion.

Table 1: Increasing size and budget at Baragwanath, 1963–78 (data from *Hospital and Nursing Yearbook 1964–1980*)

Years	Estimated patient numbers			Total maintenance expenditure	Patient days	Unit cost per patient day[14]	Unit cost per patient day in real terms[15]
	No. of beds	Inpatients	Outpatients & casualty				
1963	–	–	–	3 144 719	1 000 947	R3,14	R2,99
1964	2 128	–	–	–	–	–	–
1965	–	–	–	–	–	–	–
1965/6	–	–	–	3 916 277	958 973	R4,08	R3,79
1966/7	2 347	–	–	4 337 068	1 001 770	R4,32	R3,73
1968	–	76 974	739 749	5 379 884	1 281 596	R4,20	R3,44
1969	–	–	–	6 304 248	988 024	R6,38	R5,05
1970	2 361	–	–	–	–	–	–
1971/2				8 525 485	1 164 820	R7,32	R5,27
1972/3	2 688	77 710	868 352	9 007 387	1 165 573	R7,73	R5,23
1974	–	–	–	–	–	–	–
1975	–	–	–	11 335 890	856 643	R13,23	R6,50
1976[16]	–	–	–	20 969 624	829 030	R25,29	R11,19
1977	–	99 170	980 038	23 916 822	846 926	R28,24	R11,24
1978	–	97 751	981 021	25 833 138	839 919	R30,75	R11,01
1978/9	2 714	96 794	1 100 617	29 882 148	802 348	R37,24	R13,34

While the hospital was expanding there were also other changes in Soweto. By the 1970s, urban townships were increasingly becoming the sites of urban control. During this decade the Non-European Affairs Department (NEAD) of the Johannesburg City Council was replaced by the Bantu Affairs Administration Boards (BAABs), which acted as a form of segregated local government and were answerable to the national government. These changes saw a marked decline in services, including health services, which the city council had previously rendered to the urban African community in places like Soweto.[17]

Soweto was also in upheaval in the aftermath of the uprising led by the township's school students on 16 June 1976. Baragwanath was the largest institution in Soweto and there was pressure on the hospital to allow it to be used as a military base. Doctors tell stories of the hospital being surrounded by police and police vehicles. Government attention focused on the hospital was therefore military, not medical.

Yet on the more general health front, this was also an era in which the National Party government was more active in health care. In the early 1970s, it took over the running of hospitals for patients suffering from infectious diseases which had previously been run by local authorities. Later in the decade, the passage of the new Health Act No. 63 of 1977 set about redefining and redistributing the roles of different sectors while maintaining the three-tier system where the national, provincial and local authorities each oversaw different aspects of health care. After these changes, the provinces continued to oversee general hospital services. They were empowered by provincial ordinances to appoint all provincial personnel and to maintain hospitals and other health services. Significantly, following the passage of the new Health Act provincial services were becoming more identified with curative health services – and thus hospitals – while local authorities focused attention on hygiene and sanitation. The national government was charged with safeguarding and promoting public and community health, including the provision of psychiatric care, treatment of infectious disease, laboratory work and provision of district surgeons.

With this Act came renewed calls for more adequate clinic facilities and medical services in the townships. In Soweto, developments included the establishment of a more comprehensive ambulance service and the appointment of the first medical officer of health specifically for Soweto. By 1980, the number of clinics in Soweto had grown to nineteen – eleven controlled by the Johannesburg City Council and eight under the supervision of the province and linked to Baragwanath.

Another change that directly affected Baragwanath was the shift to a black hospital board. Although it received some media coverage,[18] this change went almost unnoticed among the staff. One doctor said to me: 'What hospital board? I had no idea such a beast existed!'. This response is not surprising. The board had, primarily, an advisory capacity. One of its major roles was attempting to keep open the lines of communication between the hospital and the Soweto community. It also dealt with the occasional inspection, the hospital choir and the arrangement of Christmas parties. The day-to-day running of the hospital remained with the superintendent and his various assistants and deputies.

During the 1980s, Soweto saw no fewer than nine health service providers or bureaucracies providing services in different, and sometimes overlapping, areas. The national Department of Health and Welfare and the TPA's Department of Hospital Services operated throughout Soweto. The Johannesburg City Health Department, the Health Department of the Transvaal Board for the Development of Peri-Urban Areas and the Health Department of Roodepoort operated in different areas of the township and provided local-level services. A number of other departments were also linked to health services: the Soweto Community Council, the Diep-Meadow Community Council, the Dobsonville Community Council and the West Rand Administration Board which, from the early 1970s, took over the daily administration of Soweto from the Non-European Affairs Department of the Johannesburg City Council. The country as a whole had fourteen overlapping bureaucracies and health ministries. The ten 'homelands' each had their own ministries of health and there were four ministries, one for each race group and one general affairs, within the rest of South Africa. These were further fragmented into eighteen separate health administrations and complemented by a number of 'welfare' organisations which functioned outside the purview of the state.

There is an almost total lack of communication and coordination between the different providers of health care. Under the present system of health services organisation with its multiple lines of authority it is extremely difficult to improve this situation and to co-ordinate the efforts of health workers in any one area.[19]

The Health Act had little chance to make a substantial difference in Soweto or at Baragwanath because the health services were already stretched too thin and had too little money. By the late 1970s, Baragwanath had entered into a phase of outrageous overcrowding, dismal conditions and a chronic lack of funding. However, especially before 1977, the overlapping health authorities gave the institution, or individuals within the institution, a space in which they could navigate, champion certain projects and develop new areas of clinical practice and interest.

Doctors and hospital administrators could also use personal networks to gain access to supplies, additional staff or money for research and equipment. The way the system functioned meant that there were various levels to which the hospital administration could apply for funding or equipment. Chris van den Heever tells of how he could seek a piece of laboratory equipment from the local city council, the TPA and – in some cases – central government. Sometimes he was turned down by all three but at other times he found his request fitted within the ambit of each level of government and he could end up with three of the same piece of equipment. But anecdotes are also told of the TPA's seemingly arbitrary decisions regarding what equipment should or should not be purchased. Asher Dubb, speaking years later, recalled that: 'Sometimes you would order equipment and only half would come.' In other cases, medical staff used their personal connections. André Giraud admitted that he would often ask friends in private practice to give him surgical implements that he could not get at the hospital.

Sometimes the doctors played the system by publicly embarrassing the administration. Yet, as Haroon Saloojee explained, this could also have negative consequences:

> I have often had to ask the question of is it worth embarrassing the administration into providing something, compared to the counter effect, where you take away the confidence in the hospital ... and that then undermines your patients' confidence in the integrity of the whole system.

Chris van den Heever has pointed to a different form of 'playing the system' by Baragwanath's superintendents. Superintendents had to balance the needs of their political bosses, their own positions and hospital requirements, and being caught between these different masters could have some advantages because it 'also meant that you could always play the political game'. He suggests that an important part of this was not alienating the political officials and explains that Isadore Frack, superintendent during the 1960s, was unsuccessful because 'he had to deal with the aftermath of Sharpeville, and he did go one step too far and got himself fired. He had daily press conferences and this embarrassed the minister'.

Unlike Frack, former superintendents Van den Heever and Beukes were careful not to embarrass the political administration with which, being Afrikaners, they had good relationships. Beukes claims that he was also able to communicate with and gain the trust of youth, during the days following the 1976 uprisings, through a series of notes between himself and youth leaders. He was then able to use his position, as someone trusted by both sides, to negotiate for the youth to enter the hospital to visit their injured friends at a particular time, not stopped by the police and army who surrounded the hospital. In exchange, the students would not storm the hospital and would not destroy hospital property or ambulances.[20]

Chris van den Heever recalled that in order to maintain a good relationship with his political bosses (which would ultimately benefit the hospital) he would sometimes have to cooperate with the security forces but he did so in a way that would not overly compromise the hospital. He explained that:

the security police were always trying to find sources of information. It became obvious after we had the 1985 strike. I suddenly had this guy who had been part of the army and had resigned, he had just gone from a uniform into a *spook* [literally 'ghost', but in this context 'spy'] and I could see the sort of questions he was asking, he was busy pumping information so I gave him information, information that I knew they already had.

Van den Heever also used his good relations with the provincial authorities in order to gain their support for the improvement of conditions at the hospital. One such case occurred during the 1980s:

Because of the media frenzy about all of the people on the floor here, it became embarrassing to government. So we had a contingent of ministers coming to visit Bara to see for themselves together with the provincial administration: the administrator, the MEC for health and all the main role players ... we marched them through the wards and they saw for themselves. Then they came for lunch ... and we made sure that there was plenty of the right stuff, so we plied them with wine from the Cape and the best whisky from Scotland and the like. We had the ministers and the leader of the National Party in the Transvaal and that sort of contingent, we are talking senior cabinet ministers. When we got to the end of the meal, the administrator said, 'Well, gentlemen, what are we going to do to improve conditions' – he was ready to talk.

Finally, Van den Heever also attempted to use the media to promote a positive image of the hospital.

... it was always my philosophy that I wanted to see my hospital's name in the paper every day. Good or bad. Because then you remain in the public eye, you remain focused, a bad story can always have a good outcome if you use it constructively. If you get told your wards look terrible, they are not painted and there is a hole in the roof, you say yes, sure it is like that, but let us look at the reasons for this. You are a taxpayer and I am a taxpayer and the taxpayers' money has to go into this and there is just not enough taxpayers' money to go into this and cover all these. You can always put a slant to it and as long as the hospitals name is there everyday you can use it to get the powers that be to better things here.

Pressure from the newspapers and the public support their reports garnered had an important effect in bringing resources to the hospital. The public nature of reports put pressure on the hospital authorities to provide specific resources. They also encouraged private donations which included paint, bedding and even medical equipment.

The medical profession's control of important aspects of the hospital also meant that segregation was never achieved as completely in medicine as it was in other areas of life in South Africa such as education. Two factors could be at play here. First, the maintenance of professional control, specialist knowledge and medical professionalism and the realities of medical training in South Africa meant that there was always some racial integration at different levels. Second, there was never a department analogous to that of Bantu Education charged with the oversight of segregation in the medical sector.

The fragmented layers of political responsibility for health had the benefit of providing a space in which the practice of medicine could take priority over segregation.

Baragwanath as an apartheid teaching hospital: The role of Wits

Baragwanath was the teaching hospital for the University of the Witwatersrand, a status that deeply affected its character and capacity to provide effective medical care. The links to the university meant that the hospital could provide cutting-edge treatment and support internationally recognised research. At the same time, the link between Baragwanath's doctors and Wits medical school meant that doctors at Baragwanath were not practising in total isolation. Many doctors, nurses, hospital administrators and, indeed, national and provincial governments stressed the sophisticated and advanced medical specialisation that was available to the black population at Baragwanath. Senior Baragwanath doctors would be called to the Johannesburg General Hospital to perform certain procedures, while others moved between the academic hospitals. The access to an unusually large patient load with a variety of chronic and acute ailments, as well as substantial links to the Wits medical school, meant that despite the frustrations and poor conditions at the hospital Baragwanath offered an unrivalled experience to those who worked there. As a result, a number of clinicians and researchers whose work was widely recognised chose to stay at Baragwanath. There was also a very much darker side of the relationship between the university and the hospital, one which was rooted in the structural inequality of apartheid.

The link between the university and the hospital dates back to the immediate post-war period. Wits played an influential role in attracting staff for Baragwanath's wards and would also hold academic appointments at the university. A lack of appropriately trained South African doctors meant that the university had to recruit the academic staff it needed from abroad, especially from the United Kingdom.

Conditions in post-war Britain were not ideal. Demobilised doctors found it difficult to find jobs after their return to the United Kingdom from service in the armed forces. Letters to the *British Medical Journal* from the period suggest this problem was particularly acute for those whose wartime training was not recognised as sufficient to practise in the post-war hospital system.[21] In addition, it was an uncertain time in the British medical world as the Labour government planned to take control of the medical services, following the beginning of the National Health Service (NHS) in July 1948. The salaries offered in South Africa were comparable to those in the United Kingdom, especially in light of the fact that in the decade leading up to the introduction of the NHS it was argued that doctors' salaries had failed to respond to the increasing cost of living in the United Kingdom. South Africa was thus a viable economic destination for British doctors.

Recognising that the new hospital might offer attractive opportunities to British doctors, Wits placed advertisements in the *British Medical Journal* and sent a recruiter to the UK. The man chosen for the job was Jack Douglas, former senior surgeon at the Johannesburg Hospital. These strategies brought to Baragwanath an international contingent of just under a dozen specialists, many of whom gathered in London and made the passage to South Africa together on a Union Castle Line ship.[22]

At the same time the national government and provincial authorities were debating Baragwanath's function in the training of black doctors and the role these doctors might play in staffing the hospital. Wits was also drawn into the discussions. Prior to the war, the small number of black doctors who practised in South Africa had, with very few exceptions, trained overseas.[23] During the war this was no longer possible and increasing pressure was put on local institutions to offer medical training. The University of Cape Town (UCT) began accepting coloured and Indian students, but not black students – allegedly because of a lack of clinical facilities for them at Groote Schuur Hospital. Almost a decade later, in 1951, the Natal Medical School opened, with an intake of about forty black students who followed a seven-year curriculum rather than the six years undertaken by white students. In 1941, Wits had become an 'open university' with the admission of black students to the medical school for the clinical years. Black students were, however, never really welcome at Wits, and by the end of the war university officials were arguing for the creation of a separate medical college for the training of black students to be based at Baragwanath.[24]

This was not to be. The university failed to gain governmental support for the idea and was left to train black medical students at its main campus. Clinical training was done at black hospitals. A number of obstacles meant that the number of black doctors who graduated remained low. Even before the implementation of Bantu Education in 1953, most black youth were subjected to an inferior education system and few had the qualifications to enter medical school. Further obstacles were also introduced. During the early 1940s a rule was introduced (with the strong support of Humphrey Raikes, Wits's principal) preventing black students from entering medical school until they had completed a first degree at the South African Native College, Fort Hare.[25] This stipulation increased the cost, time and difficulty of medical training. The Extension of Universities Act in 1959 demanded that black students apply for ministerial approval (which was seldom forthcoming) for admission to a 'white' university such as Wits. A number of faculty, students and administrators at Wits strongly opposed this legislation, but to no avail.

Even when black students were given permission to attend 'white' universities they faced an extraordinary degree of discrimination and humiliation. At Wits there was, supposedly, academic integration but social segregation. In reality, facilities at the university and at training hospitals such as Baragwanath were segregated – and vastly unequal. Black students were barred from attending post-mortems conducted on white bodies. They would have to wait outside until the organs were removed, as they were allowed to view the organs but not the body of a white person. In many cases, when black students were allowed into 'European' hospitals, they were not allowed to wear their white coats or stethoscopes and had to enter the hospital through a separate back entrance.[26]

Even once black medical students had navigated these hurdles, they could not immediately be employed at a hospital such as Baragwanath. Students who had entered medical training on a government scholarship, as many black students did, were obliged to work among their 'own people' in the rural areas for a number of years.

This resulted in the contradictory situation where some at Baragwanath and at Wits wanted and needed more black doctors, and where there were black students who wanted to apply, and yet government and elements within the Wits administration were reluctant to increase the number of black medical students admitted. Between the mid-1940s and the 1980s the number of black medical students at Wits and the number of black doctors at Baragwanath remained remarkably low. In 1945 there were eighty-two black medical students at Wits: forty-six Indians, thirty-three Africans and three coloured. Changes to the system of admissions to the medical school produced a sharp rise in the number of black enrolments at Wits in 1952 but the increase was short-lived and in the following year a quota system was introduced which limited admission to eight black students in the first year and twelve in the second. By 1959 numbers of black medical graduates were climbing slightly again and there were eighty-four black medical graduates from Wits in that year.[27] During the 1960s and 1970s black medical students constituted, on average, less than ten per cent of Wits classes.[28] More broadly, between 1968 and 1977, an average of three per cent of South Africa's medical graduates were black.[29] In 1969 there were only thirty black doctors working within the TPA structures which employed over a thousand white doctors.[30] The opening of the Medical University of South Africa (Medunsa), established in 1976 specifically to train black medical personnel, led to an increased number of black doctors in the 1980s. In the late 1970s, ministerial permission was granted to increase the number of black medical students at 'white' universities, and in 1985 the stumbling block of black students having to obtain ministerial approval to attend these universities was removed. Between 1977 and 1988 the percentage of black medical students at Wits – in all years – rose from 8.9 to 28.9.[31]

The actual numbers of black doctors at Baragwanath are difficult to obtain from the existing records. The first black interns began at Baragwanath in 1952 and full-time black doctors began working at Baragwanath in the mid-1950s.[32] Interviewed in 2004, David Blumsohn remembered that when he was an intern at Baragwanath in 1955 there 'were only two black doctors and a couple of Indian doctors'. An anonymous and undated report suggests that of the 217 doctors in full-time service at Baragwanath in 1969, twenty were black.[33] By the end of the 1970s black doctors made up only five percent of Baragwanath's 492 medical posts.[34] In 1986, out of a total of almost 500 doctors, there were only fifteen black doctors and a handful of part-time black consultants on Baragwanath's staff.

Most black medical graduates went immediately into private practice. The reasons, while complex, were essentially the result of apartheid medicine. Black doctors at public institutions were paid less than their white counterparts and were entitled to less leave. At Baragwanath black doctors ate in prefabricated buildings without the comforts of the white tearooms, and they were excluded from privileges such as the travel allowances given to Baragwanath's white staff in the early 1970s. Private practice, on the other hand, offered some degree of freedom and a respite from the direct racism doctors confronted within the apartheid system.[35]

Yet individual doctors, black and white, were able to practise ethical and quality medicine at Baragwanath. They were able to protect victims of torture, offer world-class medical treatments and Baragwanath doctors also never practised in total isolation because of the hospitals links to the medical school at Wits.

Wits and Baragwanath: Clinical and academic reasons for being at Baragwanath

There are great advantages [in being at Baragwanath]. At that time, if you were interested in academic surgery or medicine and wanted a full medical life you could do very well in the public health system and at Bara. There you had a massive patient load and you would have lots of teaching and the possibility for research and so the full timer could work a full life.

With these words Buddy Lawson, who was a surgeon at Baragwanath from 1970 to 1991, captured in a 2004 interview the essence of the academic and clinical motivations for his association with Baragwanath. He stressed the unparalleled opportunities the hospital was seen to offer despite its location and lack of resources.

Discussions about the clinical work done at Baragwanath highlight one of the central contradictions at the hospital. While the hospital was overcrowded and underfunded, it was also an urban academic hospital where doctors had access to many of the latest, sophisticated technologies. Thus, although patients often lacked basic care, linen or even a bed, it was possible for the doctors at Baragwanath to advance themselves professionally and perform complex medical procedures.

For many Baragwanath doctors, the link to and support from the Wits medical school provided the impetus for academic medicine, brought facilities to the hospital and led to a concern with academic standards and thus standards of care. For Reg Broekman, who qualified in the early 1970s and who has spent much of the last two decades as a hospital administrator, the value of the link between the hospital and the medical school is clear. 'It is a teaching hospital and it makes all the difference in the world to Bara. If you want to see chaos, deregister it as a teaching hospital and then there would be no particular reason for anybody to be there.' A similar point is made by Haroon Saloojee who qualified in the late 1970s:

> There is no doubt about it that if you excluded that link that would make the Bara experience a less exciting and less enticing alternative. So what did the academic link mean? I think it meant that you had a calibre of clinicians and other people who represented excellence. That is what you wanted to be surrounded by as young doctors or as peers.

Saloojee points to the importance of the link to the medical school in maintaining the calibre of experts with whom young doctors, interns and registers want to work. Thus, it was not unusual to hear doctors say, as did Desmond Pantanowitz: 'After I qualified I went to work at Bara with Prof Lawson for ten years, he was the best surgeon around and *the* person to learn from'. This cycle also created a sense that Baragwanath was a worthwhile place to be and a place where one could learn. Max Price, dean of the Medical Faculty at Wits between 1996 and 2006, explained his choice to do his internship at Baragwanath in 1977 as follows:

> There were many consultants and leading physicians there, especially physicians, who seemed in my mind to have as much status as the heads from JHB and the other hospitals ... The people I remember were Leo Schamroth, who was the head of cardiology, Asher Dubb, and Lawson was the head of surgery, so I thought it was a good hospital and a good training hospital. I chose to do my internship there ... I thought it was the place I could get the best teaching because the teachers were good there.

Many white Wits doctors who had a choice of hospitals did their internships at Baragwanath where they thought they would receive the best training and treat a wide variety of interesting and extreme pathology. There was something else which drew young doctors to Baragwanath for their internships: the mythology that had been built up about the hospital within Wits and medical services more generally. The legendary Bara spirit excited students who wanted to be part of the special and unique medicine that was said to be practised there.

The perception that Baragwanath provided first-rate training has been challenged, most recently by the Truth and Reconciliation Commission and by the Internal Reconciliation Commission (IRC) held by the Wits Faculty of Medicine.[36] A number of black doctors pointed out that they were denied the choices that white medical students had because they were confined to the black hospitals where they did not have access to the same range of experiences and facilities. They argued that the teaching they had access to was unequal and inferior. Role models for black doctors were lacking and many black students felt that they did not get the same type of mentoring that white students got from senior staff.[37]

For many hospital staff the teaching component of academic medicine was most important. Moira Russell, a graduate in obstetrics and gynaecology of Glasgow University came to Baragwanath 'to gain experience' in 1971, and remained for twenty-seven years. She noted that 'most medical staff found the student teaching component of our jobs to be stimulating, challenging and rewarding'.[38] Ken Huddle, who was appointed as head of the Department of Medicine at Baragwanath in 1990 but whose involvement with the hospital dates back to his year as an intern in 1975, echoed this sentiment in an interview when he stressed that: 'Teaching keeps you on your toes and keeps you current, that whole environment is very positive'. For others, like Buddy Lawson, it was more than just rewarding, it was an essential component of a 'full medical life'.

Some also stressed the aspects of teaching that were unique to Baragwanath. Huddle, for example, explained that 'here people are prepared to teach, we still teach a lot around the bedside which is a dying art. That attracts people here, and it is a different experience ... it is the glue that keeps people here, the excitement of training new doctors to provide good services for our patients'.

The relationship between the medical school and the hospital also had material advantages because it brought technologies that were employed as teaching tools to the hospital. For example, in the late 1970s the medical school arranged for the TPA to purchase the province's first whole-body scanner for Baragwanath. Cutting-edge technology and implements were also made available to the surgical team for teaching and in order for them to carry out new research.[39] This was also part of the broader paradox of Baragwanath – while the majority of patients were suffering from diseases connected to poverty and the hospital was often unable to provide basic care, some patients were being treated with sophisticated, expensive equipment.

For a number of doctors, Baragwanath's location opened opportunities for research. Yet, its existence as one of the few places where the Soweto population could access biomedical health care meant that doctors faced an ever-increasing patient load that threatened to subsume academic research. David Blumsohn felt that 'because the patient care has overwhelmed us all these years our teaching is included in our treating people and research has always taken a second back seat'. Responses to the 1955 Commission of Enquiry into Medical Research suggest that this might have been the case from as early as the mid-1950s.[40] One surgeon, complaining of the premature discharge of patients owing to the bed shortage and the difficulties of follow-up with outpatients, further noted that 'the excessive amount of routine ward work is reflected in the additional strain thrown on the radiological and pathological services – essential departments in any research project. In essence the pressure of routine and administrative duties in a busy, overcrowded hospital provides all too little opportunity for research'.[41]

Some doctors clearly felt the pressure of the patient loads, and research did slow down, especially from the 1980s. Those interviewed, however, continued to express a pride in the new techniques and skills they introduced and the types of research they could engage in. Indeed, senior Baragwanath doctors such as Giraud and Hunt were called to the Johannesburg General Hospital to perform certain procedures, while others moved between the academic hospitals.[42]

The struggle for control over nursing at Baragwanath Hospital

The roots of training black nurses to serve in a western hospital setting in South Africa date back to the early 1900s. These early efforts were slow and marred by conflicts over who should pay for the training, arguments over the suitability of black candidates for training as nurses, the small and isolated nature of many of the training schools and the fact that only a small number of black women came forward to be trained.[43] However, by the 1930s other factors came into play. The large-scale construction of hospitals, as well as a growing demand for district and other health-care services available to Africans in the urban and rural areas meant that more nurses were needed.[44] Increasing pressure on the government to meet this demand resulted in the decision by the Department of Native Affairs to subsidise the training of black nurses at mission institutes from the early 1930s.[45] However, this did not go far enough. In 1942, the Smit Committee urged that 'facilities for the training of native nurses and midwives should be increased by every possible means'. Shortly thereafter the Gluckman Commission again emphasised the chronic shortage of nurses.

The demand for the government to provide adequate training for black nurses, especially during the 1940s, was also linked to the pressure to train black doctors. Black ward sisters would be vital if hospitals such as Baragwanath were to train black medical students. The main reason for this was the desire to avoid a situation where black interns, registrars or doctors would give instructions to white ward sisters.[46] It is ironic that the acceptance of black nurses and the expansion of a professional occupation for black women was the result of an attempt to introduce stricter racial segregation and stratification.

The training of black nurses to care for black patients was deeply intertwined with a long and complex deliberation about race. Calls to train black nurses during the preceding decades were met with fears about the intimate contact that might result between white nurses and black patients, concerns about the competency of Africans to be trained as nurses and anxiety about the threat black nurses might become on the job market. By the 1950s it seems as if it was the disquiet over issues of race that precipitated a significant increase in the training of black nurses and the move to replace all white nurses serving at black hospitals with black nurses. The formidable Charlotte Searle, who was at the time the director of Nursing Service in Transvaal Provincial Administration, was told that she 'must take steps forthwith to prepare the Bantu nurse in as short a period as possible and by whatever means she and the matrons in the service found appropriate to take over the responsibility for running all the nursing services in the non-white health services'.[47]

Another important factor in advancing the training of black nurses was the policy of separate development, the main ideological reason for the government's focus on the increased provision of training facilities for black nurses and the rapid promotion of these nurses into senior positions at black hospitals. The government saw this process as important because trained nurses were needed in the Bantustans if they were to function as separate entities. At the same time, nurses were seen as part of an African elite that could be coopted into the administration of the Bantustans.

Against this background, the new secular training colleges for black nurses opened in the Transvaal. In 1939, the Pretoria Hospital, under the Transvaal Provincial Administration, had already been registered as a training hospital for black nurses. Shortly thereafter Wits introduced a diploma course which was open to both white and black students, but applicants required a matriculation certificate and two years' post-basic experience to be admitted – and few black students had the entry qualifications. The lack of qualifications was a major stumbling block because many black women saw nursing as a high-status career. Indeed, although nursing and teaching were not the only professional jobs available to black women until the birth of a democratic South Africa in 1994, they were by far the most commonplace. Most of the black women entering nursing, at least in the early years, were trained in a mission setting. This will be discussed in Chapter 5.

The Non-European Hospital in Johannesburg followed suit and began training black nurses in 1940. The hospital, which did not demand such stringent qualifications for entrance, was more successful than the universities in training black nurses. It appointed its first three black staff nurses in 1942 and its first black ward sister in January 1948 – four months before the opening of Baragwanath Hospital.[48] Despite these developments, and the Non-European Hospital's attempts to build up extra staff in anticipation of the opening of Baragwanath, it was foreseen, even in the hospital's early years, that many more nurses would be needed. Thus, in October 1947 the Baragwanath Nursing College was opened with a class of fifty-seven students under the supervision of Mrs GA MacGillivray and Miss Margaret Burnett, who had recently retired from her post as deputy matron at the Johannesburg Hospital.[49] In 1948, the black nursing students from the Johannesburg Hospital, together with three white tutors, were moved to Baragwanath, bringing the number of students at the hospital up to 240.[50]

This was hardly a sufficient nursing staff for the rapidly expanding Baragwanath in its civilian guise. The question of where to train black nurses and who should control their training and professional conduct brought Baragwanath Hospital, Wits, the TPA and two of the nursing governing bodies, the South African Nursing Association (SANA) and the South African Nursing Council (SANC), into a complex administrative web.

From the earliest discussions about the conversion of the hospital to civilian use there was a call by those overseeing the transformation for the establishment of a nursing college for black nurses at the hospital. Between

1940 and 1990, Baragwanath Nursing College developed into one of the largest training colleges for black nurses in South Africa. When the hospital opened as a civilian hospital in 1948, the nursing staff complement was made up of three white matrons, thirty-three white sisters, two black sisters and 118 black staff nurses.[51] By the 1950s the hospital was receiving between 2 000 and 3 000 applications for an estimated 250 to 300 positions at the training college.[52] Three decades later, the new Baragwanath College of Nursing, which could accommodate 1 500 students per year, had opened, but this went only part of the way towards meeting the demand for places because by this time Baragwanath was receiving between 20 000 and 30 000 applications per year. While many of these applications were not complete and many applicants did not meet the stringent educational requirements to enter nurse training, these figures point to the limited employment opportunities open to black women in South Africa at that time. They also suggest why a sense of privilege and common professional identity formed among those who were accepted, even as the backgrounds from which the candidates were drawn became more diverse.

A far larger number of nursing students entered training at the Baragwanath Nursing College than graduated. Despite stringent entrance requirements there was a high dropout rate. Lydia Hebestreit, lecturer at the college from 1958 and principal of the college between 1960 to 1966, suggests that the key reasons for non-completion were pregnancy, difficulty in adjusting to the hospital environment and failure in exams due to lack of language ability. By one estimate, as many as sixty per cent of the nurses accepted into training did not complete the course in the late 1960s.[53] Jane McLarty, Baragwanath's chief matron, unlike many of her peers, blamed the high rate of failure on conditions within the hospital and on the structure of training, rather than on the unsuitability of black nurses. McLarty introduced a pre-nursing course,[54] a Baragwanath version of the 'cadets' programme that the provincial administration introduced in 1952. It ran for between one and six months and focused on assisting nurses to adapt to the urban environment and become accustomed to the protocols of the nursing school.[55] Young recruits were taught not only English-language skills, mathematics and biology but also social sciences (focusing on the ethics and history of nursing). While the programme at Baragwanath carried on into the next decade with mixed success, 'cadets' was discontinued in 1960 when the TPA ceased to perceive it as useful because of general social changes among Africans.[56]

During the 1950s universities such as Wits became another thread in the web of nurses training – but one which, at this stage, had only a minor effect on Baragwanath Hospital. Basic nursing training was incorporated into universities. As in much of the rest of the world, South African nursing leaders attempted to increase the status of nurses by moving courses to university settings and lengthening the duration of training with the thought that this would attract candidates from better backgrounds. In the context of apartheid South Africa, as Marks has argued, this was a deliberate response to the increasing numbers of black nurses moving into positions of power, especially at hospitals which catered for black patients.[57] Although the university nursing programmes were not segregated, black nurses faced the same obstacles as black doctors in trying to gain access to universities such as Wits. It was only in November 1985 that Mr Andrew Chiloane became the first black student to successfully complete the BSc Nursing degree at Wits.[58]

Nursing education at Wits and Baragwanath did, however, have other interesting connections. The first full-time senior lecturer in the new Wits BSc degree was Lydia Hebestreit. She came to Wits in 1969, from Baragwanath Nursing College where she had served as a lecturer and then principal from 1958 to 1966. One of her primary tasks was to develop and shape the new Wits degree. However, she was in the position for hardly a year when she resigned to return to Baragwanath and take up the post of director of nursing. Her successor, Shirley Williamson, speculates that Hebestreit left Wits not only to return to a setting which she found challenging but that she was also frustrated at Wits because she felt that she was not getting the support she needed to get the nursing department started. The integration of nursing training into the university system further enhanced the educational value of the degree and status of black women. Just as many nurses became key leaders in the struggle against apartheid, many former nurses took on important jobs within the university administration after the end of apartheid.

While Wits and the Baragwanath College were training nursing students, it was the SANC and SANA which controlled – at least in theory – the professional aspects of nursing. White nurses were in dominant positions in these nursing structures and hierarchies, and privileged by the legislation. In the early 1930s, the South African Trained Nurses Association was made up of and represented white nurses, while black nurses were members of the Bantu Trained Nurses Association, which was formed in 1932. This division lasted until 1944, when Act 45 of 1944 created the South African Nursing

Association (SANA) which superseded all existing organisations. The new association was, in theory at least, open to all nurses regardless of race. All nurses had the right to vote and be elected to the South African Nursing Council (SANC), nursing's governing body. This Act was passed when the number of black nurses was relatively small and when white nurses clearly dominated the association.[59] As the numbers began to shift towards the end of the following decade, legislation was changed to allow only whites to serve on the SANC and to place qualified nurses on different registers. The reaction to the latter decision was swift and momentous (as I will discuss in Chapter 5) but despite this action the segregated nature of nursing in South Africa remained unchanged.[60]

For most of the apartheid period black, coloured and Indian nurses were represented by segregated advisory boards and a committee of elected black, coloured and Indian nurses which advised the SANC on matters affecting nurses of each of their race groups. In effect this gave black nurses only indirect representation and kept the *status quo* very much as it had been when whites represented them. The boards were done away with in 1978 and white dominance of the SANA and the SANC became more entrenched even as the number of black nurses grew.

When Baragwanath nurses were questioned about these organisations, many were dismissive. Annah Montso, who began her training at Coronation Hospital in 1955, suggested that she was 'just a member. We were expected to be members of the nursing council'. When asked if the SANA or the SANC did anything for the nurses, she replied: 'Not that I know of'. Other nurses suggested that the council could help with very specific issues such as disciplinary hearings or access to lawyers. The body was also perceived as instrumental in making rules. One nurse said: 'We used to be just members. They were making rules for us; the nurse must behave like this, the nurse must dress like this and like that. It would just come from up there, coming down to us that this is what is expected so we were not very much in contact with them'. In Durban in the 1970s, Angela Cheater found that many of the nurses she interviewed regarded the SANA as a 'stooge' organisation that did not serve the needs of the black nurses.[61] Similarly, Maggie Resha showed that some black nurses perceived that the SANA was not looking after their interests, while 'their subscriptions continued to fatten the coffers of the association. Requests to act on their behalf lead to the doors being slammed in their faces'.[62] The *South African Nursing Journal* advertised meetings of the Unity

Branch of the Johannesburg SANA, which took place monthly at Baragwanath throughout the period under discussion, yet none of the nurses I interviewed stressed these meetings as being important to them.

The white nursing administrators at Baragwanath were involved in, and often served on, the SANC. McLarty was the first president of SANA and served from 1944 to 1946. She remained an influential member of the SANC and served as vice-chair in 1975, using this position to fight for the rights of black nurses and for their right to take the same exams and remain registered in the same organisation as white nurses.[63] She was also for many years the secretary for the non-European group of the Witwatersrand Branch of SANA.

White nurses remained in control of the statutory nursing body and of the profession throughout the apartheid period, although black nurses were gradually given more authority and responsibility at black hospitals. However, black nurses never had authority over white nurses and in many cases white nurses remained in a supervisory role at hospitals like Baragwanath until well into the 1980s. While black nurses were taking on supervisory roles at hospitals such as Baragwanath; the Wits Department of Nursing Education assumed responsibility for nurses training at the Baragwanath College. In June 1982, the national Department of Health and Welfare agreed to the integration of nursing education into the university system. This integration became obligatory in 1985 and meant that nursing education was finally separated from the nursing service.[64] Rather than being subordinated to the hospitals, nursing colleges became autonomous units in 1986. In practice this meant that colleges were controlled by their own councils and senates. They had their own budgets, conducted their own academic education (in most cases a four-year integrated diploma course leading to nursing registration) and set their own examinations.[65] The colleges were, however, under the academic guardianship of the universities. The Department of Nursing at Wits thus became responsible for the monitoring and controlling of standards at BG Alexander Nursing College and the Baragwanath Nursing College, as well as the nursing college at the University of Bophuthatswana in Mafikeng. The Wits Department was also responsible for inspecting the colleges, representing them on the university's senate, and moderating their examinations.

In nursing, as in all other aspects of the hospitals' administration and functioning, two factors stand out: firstly, the pervasive influence of apartheid; and secondly, the multiple layers of institutions and bodies involved in the running of the hospital. Yet amid this complex structure Baragwanath was able to form its own identity.

Endnotes

1   J De Beer (1976) 'A Forward View of Health Services in South Africa', *South African Medical Journal* 50:11, March, pp. 431–2.

2   HCJ Van Rensburg, A Fourie and E Pretorius (1992) *Health Care in South Africa: Structure and Dynamics*. Pretoria: Academica: 236.

3   The Bantustans were areas in which Africans were to become self-governing and eventually independent. The word 'Bantustan' was in vogue during the Verwoerdian era and later changed to 'homelands' or 'self-governing states'.

4   TG Mashaba (1995) *Rising to the Challenge of Change: A History of Black Nursing in South Africa*. Cape Town: Juta, p. 58.

5   'Baragwanath is Proud of Record', *The Star*, 1 May 1969 cites the administrator of the Transvaal, Mr SGJ van Niekerk, as saying that '[n]on-white staff at Baragwanath Hospital will be given increasing responsibility in running the hospital'.

6   'Department of Nursing: The Women at the Heart of the Hospital', *Baragwanath Yearbook* 1992, p. 11; Mashaba op. cit., p. 59.

7   I Frack (1970) *Every Man Must Play a Part: The Story of a South African Doctor*. Cape Town: Purnell, p. 187; E Botha (1988) 'A Bara Person'. *Publico* 8:2, April: 12–13, p. 12.

8   I Frack (1958a) 'Guest Editorial: Baragwanath Hospital, Decennial Anniversary'. *Medical Proceedings* 4:10, May, p. 250 and 'Baragwanath – Place of Healing'. *South African Panorama* January 1967, p. 4.

9   'Miracle of Baragwanath: A Monument to Mercy', *The Star*, 29 March 1963.

10   *Hospital and Nursing Yearbook of Southern Africa*. Johannesburg, 1950–1990.

11   L Hebestreit (1969) 'Nursing Service and Education at Baragwanath Hospital'. *South African Medical Journal* 43:21, May, p. 673.

12   AW Simpson (1958) 'Nursing Services at the Baragwanath Hospital'. *Medical Proceedings* 4:10, May, p. 325; 'Baragwanath – Place of Healing' op. cit.

13   *Hospital and Nursing Yearbook* op. cit., pp. 71, 170–1.

14   Unit cost per patient day is calculated in the data set by dividing the total maintenance cost by the number of patient days.

15   I calculated unit cost per patient day in real terms by using the Consumer Price Index based on 1960 rands.

16   Hospital and Nursing Yearbook op. cit., p. 117. Budgets of most Transvaal hospitals were increased substantially this year. For instance, Coronation's went from R3 223 436 to R4 745 980 (per pat*ient from R19,28 to R27,47)*.

17   Carr op. cit., pp. 183–4.

18   For example: 'Bara Board Too New for Breakthrough', *POST*, 4 June 1980; 'Bara Gets a Blackboard', *Rand Daily Mail*, 13 December 1979; 'All-Black Hospital Board Inducted', *Rand Daily Mail*, 10 November 1979; 'Blacks to Run Hospital', *Sowetan* (nd).

19   Wilson op. cit., p. 24.

20   PJ Beukes 'The Day Hector Peterson Died, by the Soweto from Namaqualand' (unpublished manuscript c. 2005, in Beukes's possession), pp. 55–6.

21   B Moran, A Webb-Johnson and E Holland (1946) 'Correspondence: Demobilised Specialists'. *British Medical Journal* 2, July, p. 134.

22   Dubb op. cit., pp. 16–7.

23   Digby op. cit., p. 429; B Murray (1997) *Wits, The Open Years: A History of the University of the Witwatersrand*, Johannesburg, 1939–1959. Johannesburg: Wits University Press, p. 27.

24   Committee to Inquire into the Training of Natives in Medicine and Public Health (Loram Committee), UG 35–28; Murray op. cit., p. 323. On the role of the University of Natal in the training of black doctors during this period, see V Noble (2005) 'Doctors Divided: Gender, Race and Class Anomalies in the Production of Black Medical Doctors in Apartheid South Africa, 1948–1994'. University of Michigan PhD thesis.

25   Murray op.cit., pp. 28, 32; J Browde, E Jassat and P Mokhobo (1998) Internal Reconciliation Commission: Faculty of Health Sciences, University of the Witwatersrand, Summary Report, p. 3.

26   Browde et al., op. cit. and L Baldwin-Ragaven, J de Gruchy and L London (1999) *An Ambulance of the Wrong Colour: Health Professionals, Human Rights and Ethics in South Africa*. Cape Town: UCT Press.

27   Murray op. cit., pp. 131–4, 676.

28   Browde et al., op. cit., p. 4.

29   Baldwin-Ragaven et al., op. cit., p. 173.

30   *Transvaal Provincial Administration, Report of the Director of Hospital Services,* 12th report, 1969–1970, p. 1.

31   Browde et al. op. cit., pp. 10–1.

32   VH Wilson op. cit., p. 251; Digby op. cit., p. 442; Browde et al. op. cit., p. 13.

33   Bara PR Archives, 'Historical Overview of Baragwanath Hospital' (c. 1969), p. 9.

34   C van den Heever, cited in J Johnson and P Magubane (1981) *Soweto Speaks*. Johannesburg: AD Donker, p. 27.

35   Haroon Saloojee, 31 August 2004. See also WHSR, M3/40.1, IRC, JB Kimutai (1998) 'The Faculty of Health Sciences during the Apartheid Era: A Research Report Submitted to the Internal Reconciliation Commission' (unpublished paper), pp. 14–5 and T Goodman and M Price (1999) 'Using an Internal Reconciliation Commission to Facilitate Organisational Change in Post-Apartheid South Africa – The Case of Wits Health Science Faculty' (unpublished paper), p. 8.

36   The IRC was commissioned by the Wits Faculty of Health Sciences in 1997 to investigate and report on the role of the faculty and its teaching hospitals during the apartheid era. Browde et al. op. cit. See also Goodman and Price op. cit.

37   Browde et al. op. cit., pp. 16, 33; WHSR, M3/40, Box 4, Mohammed Tikly, e-mail submission to Jules Browde, June 1998, pp. 52–3; Farouk Dindar, e-mail submission to Max Price, June 1998, p. 57, KB Parbhoo, written submission to Max Price, May 1997, p. 135; *Truth and Reconciliation Commission of South Africa: Final Report* (Cape Town, 1998), Vol. 4, Chapter 5, paragraphs 58–9, 63, 65.

38   Moria Russell, letter to Simonne Horwitz, 6 April 2004.

39   See, for example, Hunt op. cit., pp. 93–103, 119–30.

40   The only doctors who expressed this view in interviews were David Blumsohn, 27 September 2004 and Ken Huddle, 3 August 2004.

41   SAB, GES 3012, 8, S Kleinot, Senior Surgeon, Memorandum, 'Baragwanath Hospital, Research', 15 March 1955. For similar sentiments see also SAB, GES 3012, 8, DWP. Lavery, Memorandum, 'Baragwanath Hospital, Department of Obstetrics and Gynaecology', 15 March 1955.

42   André Giraud, 12 July 2004; Hunt op. cit., pp. 62–3.

43   Marks (1994) op. cit., pp. 82–7; R Phillips (1938) *The Bantu in the City: A Study of Cultural Adjustment on the Witwatersrand*. Alice: Lovedale Press, p. 135; Mashaba op. cit., p. 38; H Sweet (2004) '"Wanted: 16 Nurses of the Better Educated Type": Provision of Nurses to South Africa in the Late Nineteenth and Early Twentieth Centuries'. *Nursing Inquiry* 11, p. 180.

44   Sweet and Digby op. cit., p. 112.

45   On the shortage of nurses see, for example, *Report of the Committee Appointed to Inquire into the Training of Natives in Medicine and Public Health* (Loram Committee, 1928), UG 35–28, paragraph. 9, p. 4 and par. 68, p. 20. On subsidising training, see Marks (1995) op. cit., pp. 88–9.

46   SAB, GES 1440, 466/19, 'Memo from George Gale, secretary for health to the minister of health', 6 February 1947; Marks (1995) op. cit., p. 140.

47   C Searle (1965) *The History of the Development of Nursing in South Africa*. Cape Town: Struik. Searle, *The History of the Development of Nursing*, p. 276.

48   Simpson op. cit., p. 325.

49   Bara PR Archives, History File, L Spies 'The History and Establishment of Baragwanath Hospital: A Comprehensive Overview of the Establishment of the Hospital and its History up to 1980' (unpublished paper, c. 1980), p. 3.

50   Hebestreit op. cit., p. 670. Although these are the figures most often quoted, the Tenth Anniversary of Baragwanath Non-European Hospital brochure, Johannesburg, 26 May 1958, p. 1 states that when Baragwanath opened there were 180 student nurses.

51   Simpson op. cit., cited in 'Baragwanath Turns 21', *Weekend World*, 6 May 1968; Hebestreit op. cit., p. 673.

52   EW Petersen (1958) 'African Nurse Training – Ten Years of Progress'. *Medical Proceedings* 4:10, May, p. 329.

53   Hebestreit op. cit., p. 671.

54   WHP, A2197, McLarty Papers, B1. 2(c): 'Baragwanath Hospital: Twelve Years of Progress' (c. 1960), pp. 6–7.

55   Mashaba op. cit., p. 41.

56   Hebestreit op. cit., p. 670.

57   Marks (1995) op. cit., p. 157.

58   *SA Digest*, Transhosp News, June 1986, p. 821.

59   Marks (1995) op. cit., pp. 123–5.

60   Op. cit., pp. 142–4.

61   AP Cheater (1974) 'A Marginal Elite? African Registered Nurses in Durban, South Africa'. *African Studies* 33, pp. 146, 143–58.

62   M Resha (1991) *'Mangoana O Tsoara Thipa ka Bohaleng': My Life in the Struggle*. Johannesburg: COSAW, p. 139.

63   'A Women's Journal', *The Star*, 18 December 1952; 'Obituary: In Memoriam – Jane McLarty (1893–1989)'. *Nursing RSA* 4:3, March 1989, p. 8.

64   This was done in 1985 with the passing of SANC regulation R425. All nursing colleges became associated with universities.

65   Adler Museum, Nursing Colleges, BG Alexander, History, 'History of Nursing Education at Johannesburg Hospital and BG Alexander Nursing College', unpublished, 12 May 1998 (on the occasion of the closure of the college).

Missionaries, Clinicians, Activists and Bara Boeties
The Doctors of Baragwanath Hospital

Baragwanath Hospital was a difficult place in which to work. For much of its existence, its overcrowded, understaffed wards were, in the words of one of its doctors, David Seftel, 'a cacophony of voices and sick sounds, a theatre of the bizarre and the absurd which was sometimes difficult to imagine as a place of healing rather than a carnival'. It was considered by many to be a 'backwater' hospital, often referred to disparagingly as 'that place beyond Uncle Charlie's' (the roadhouse that came to mark the end of Johannesburg and the beginning of Soweto) and spoken of as playing second fiddle to the older, more established white hospital, the Johannesburg General. Asher Dubb said that 'the medical school hierarchy was concentrated on the Johannesburg Hospital, that was seen as the flagship ... There was a perception, which I personally think was exaggerated, that Bara was the poor relation'.[1]

In contrast many Baragwanath doctors, including some world-class specialists, talked about the hospital in glowing tones. They stressed that Baragwanath was a unique and special place to work in, one that offered unparalleled opportunities for professional and personal growth. Then there were others for whom Baragwanath, and the type of medicine practised there, chimed well with their political and social identity.

Patients, pathology and physicians

Baragwanath could not rival Johannesburg General Hospital's research funding and resources. The third superintendent, WHF Kenny, who served from 1963 to 1969, put it as follows: 'Baragwanath Hospital has no research appointments and no research funds other than those private contributions gleaned by enthusiastic members of staff. There are no departmental typists and no tape recorders; records are liable to get lost.'[2] Two decades later there were still major discrepancies between resources at the two institutions. As David Seftel was later to say, 'At Jo'burg there were armies of people helping you, at Bara you had to draw blood yourself and get it 500 metres from the ward to the lab. You had to run it there and then back to your patient. This was health care on the edge where patients' survival was based upon your own physical agility as much as your mental acumen.' Despite these deficiencies, David Seftel perceived Baragwanath as an advantageous site for important medical innovations and developments, 'the classic case of ingenuity in the face of adversity. We had to work on our ... practical survival skills on a day to day basis. You had to be ingenious to make the best of a crumbling infrastructure and lack of resources and an extraordinary workload.'

World renowned electro-cardiologist and long-time head of the Baragwanath Department of Medicine, Leo Schamroth, also suggests that the hospital's uniqueness exists not despite its challenges, but because of them:

Baragwanath Hospital is in many respects unique. It is a hospital that pursues a vigorous practice and serves a very large community of underprivileged people. It embodies the utilitarian management of incredibly large numbers of sick people. And it is served by a relatively small, dedicated group of doctors who work under conditions which may euphemistically be termed 'rather trying'. I have always believed that adversity is a powerful stimulus, indeed, at times, an essential stimulus. And it is the stimulus of adversity that has produced the kind of doctor which we find at this hospital.[3]

It is difficult to judge Baragwanath's exceptionalism against other institutions, but what is important is the way ideas about the distinctive and special nature of the hospital are interwoven with the doctors' own sense of identity and purpose. For these doctors Baragwanath's difficult environment was part of its allure. A number of doctors emphasised the way they used the difficult conditions they encountered at Baragwanath to their advantage. These explanations and the heroic descriptions of how they coped within this environment served to represent their role at the hospital in a positive light. It was a justification for being there. In interviews and in their writing, doctors cast themselves not as practising in the backwaters of medicine but as developing specific skills which made the kinds of medicine they practised unique.

Baragwanath's location close to a rapidly urbanising, predominantly poor population presented advantages for clinical research. From the 1950s, the impact of urbanisation on epidemiology and the relationship between the effects of urbanisation and different parts of the body (for example the heart) was a significant focus of the research. The effects of poor nutrition, *mngomboti* (African beer) and indigenous medicines on diseases of the alimentary canal, as well as deficiency diseases like beriberi and scurvy were all subjects of investigation.[4] The Department of Paediatrics examined nutritional diseases such as marasmus, pellagra, scurvy and rickets; and the complications of diarrhoeal disorders.[5] It was Baragwanath paediatrician Alfred Altmann who revolutionised the treatment of protein malnutrition (malignant malnutrition or kwashiorkor) when he recognised that it was primarily a protein and not a vitamin deficiency syndrome.[6] These diseases were mostly related to the poor nutrition, housing and sanitation that characterised the living conditions of many urban Africans. The social determinants of health had a major influence on the patient body at Baragwanath but also shaped the doctors' research. Many doctors were politicised by their close contact with the apartheid conditions their patients had to endure and this led several of them to become activists.

One area of growing interest in the decades that followed was the effect of urbanisation and westernisation on diseases of the bowel. In the early 1970s, Cedric Bremner, for example, published a thirteen-year survey of changing patterns of disease seen at Baragwanath Hospital. He argued that the disease patterns among rural Africans changed with urbanisation. Changes in diet and lifestyle led to a significant increase in the incidence of bowel diseases such as haemorrhoids and appendicitis as well as diseases such as breast cancer.[7] Issy Segal, a well known gastroenterologist at Baragwanath, studied the development of diseases of the digestive tract in urban blacks. His work resulted in over fifty articles, mostly written during the 1970s and the 1980s,[8] and his findings, as represented in a 1979 article, suggested that certain bowel diseases – including polyps, ulcerative colitis, irritable bowel syndrome, diverticular disease, and colon cancer – remained uncommon although an increase in diverticular disease was noted. The article does, however, predict that further changes in diet will increase the prevalence of these diseases in the black population.[9]

Schamroth, author of over 300 scientific publications, seven textbooks and six monographs, was interested in how social change, especially rapid urbanisation, affected both patterns of disease and medical practice.[10] This was an interest for which there were few better research sites than Baragwanath. In 1985, looking back over a career at Baragwanath which began in 1956 and spanned three decades, Schamroth discussed some of the changing disease patterns he saw at the hospital. He noted the eradication of typhoid fever with Soweto's water-based sewerage system and hoped for the reduction of lung disease with electrification, and he went on to note the growth of new diseases in Soweto's population:

> The disease spectrum which the doctors of this hospital have to deal with is in many respects a microcosm of the turmoil, the cauldron of change, in which South Africa finds itself today ...The adverse effects of westernisation and urbanisation are also becoming apparent. Small in numbers though they may be, we are now seeing cases of the classic westernised heart attack, cases of duodenal ulcer and of ulcerative colitis. Diseases which were previously unknown in this population. We therefore not only have the function and privilege of treating and caring for these sick people but we have, in effect, a unique field laboratory where, by studying the deleterious effects of westernisation, of urbanisation on the African peoples, we can help elucidate the challenging diseases of the twentieth century.[11]

Despite numerous complaints about the conditions at Baragwanath and despite international job offers, Schamroth spent almost his entire working life at the hospital. It gave him not only the possibility for research but also the opportunity to teach and to treat a patient population in desperate need of health care. Fighting for better conditions for the patients was an important part of Schamroth's personal and political identity. Baragwanath, with all its problems, and perhaps because of them, was the only place where Schamroth could imagine himself working.

From a clinical point of view, the huge patient load has always meant that doctors could do more procedures, more often. On the tenth anniversary of the opening of the civilian hospital, the superintendent declared with some pride: 'At Baragwanath the unusual becomes commonplace, the wards often resembling living medical museums. Visiting scientists of world-fame and renown are amazed at the multiplicity and variety of disease and their manifestations, which are seldom seen outside textbooks'.[12] Another doctor, commenting two decades later on her own experience, remembered 'a Belgian elective student sitting down opposite me at lunch time one day and saying that he had seen more obstetrical complications in the labour ward that morning than he had seen in his entire obstetrics block at home!'.[13] These large numbers also played an important role in academic case studies. Reg Broekman later explained that, 'you can get more cases at Bara than you can at any other hospital, so the time that you take to do the research project is at least half if not less for case collections. So it is highly attractive from that point of view'.

A 1970s obstetrics study of 'Transverse Lie in Labour' conducted at Baragwanath, for example, had the largest series of data of any published work on this topic.[14] The huge series allowed the authors to make a number of important suggestions about the management of such cases. Similarly, a study of gallstone disease done at Baragwanath in the 1980s had what was 'probably the largest series reported in black patients'.[15] So, while the huge patient load did have some very negative effects on working at Baragwanath and on patient care, it was also one of the features mentioned by doctors that made the hospital unique.

Doctors saw a very wide range of diseases and pathology, often at far more advanced stages than seen in most white urban hospitals. Not only did the patients who received care at Baragwanath suffer from the diseases of poverty, but some patients travelled a great distance from regions where western bio-medical care was often severely lacking. Doctors knew that many of their patients had sought other health care options – especially from indigenous healers – prior to coming to the hospital, but often hid this from the doctors who tended to see indigenous healers in a negative light.[16] For example, in their 1979 article on 'The Witchdoctor and the Bowel' researched at Baragwanath, Issy Segal and Leonard Ou-Tim acknowledged that most urban Africans consult indigenous healers, but they argued that the potent effects of herbal medicines often resulted in damage to the gastrointestinal tract that could be fatal, and they suggested that at a hospital such as Baragwanath diseases which result from the ingestion of herbal medicines constitute an important facet of the disease spectrum.[17]

Consulting traditional or alternative health care providers delayed some patients coming to the hospital; others delayed because they could not afford even the minimal costs of seeking medical care in the public sector. Therefore, many waited until diseases were advanced before seeking hospital care. For many, Baragwanath became a place of last resort. The neglect of preventative medicine in the South African health care system, and at medical schools, which – at least until the 1970s – focused on tertiary health care in the hospital setting, compounded this problem.[18]

In a letter to me, Moira Russell explained that the extreme pathology was one of the things that 'made working at Bara so dynamic and challenging – just when you thought that you had "seen it all" a patient with an even rarer condition (really small print at the bottom of the textbook page) would suddenly appear.' For example, Crohn's disease was said to be nonexistent in the black South African population, yet a Baragwanath research team used the administration records of 527,048 patients to prove that this was not in fact correct.[19] A 1977 article refers to the absence of spinal stenosis in black patients[20] whereas Baragwanath doctors were able to show that among the admissions to the Orthopaedic Spinal Unit between 1983 and 1986 there were in fact a small number of these cases.[21] Bringing the possibility of this disease in black patients to the attention of the medical community was important for diagnosis, and further dispelled the myth of racial differences in disease profiles.

In addition, the nature of the hospital and its patients led to specific developments in clinical practice. '[T]he only way to achieve and maintain an acceptable quality of care' according to one doctor who worked at Baragwanath, 'is to exploit creative solutions, in order to adapt the existing infrastructure and to devise efficient clinical protocols for the benefit of the greatest number'.[22] For example, the high incidence of gastroenteritis during the 1950s led to the creation of the first paediatric drip room. The drip room consisted of rows of cots in which babies could be placed while drips were inserted into veins in their head for a rapid intake of fluid and thus hydration of the child. Babies were treated on an out-patient basis and tended by their mothers. In most cases, there was no need to admit them into already overcrowded wards. The service was copied both locally and in other parts of the developing world.[23]

Township violence was always a cause of admission to Baragwanath, notoriously on Friday and Saturday nights. Stab wounds to the spine, heart and abdomen were routinely dealt with during the 1950s and 1960s. The 1970s saw ever-increasing numbers of gunshot wounds. Blunt head trauma was also common. The growing number of motor vehicles in and around Soweto led to an increase in motor accident related trauma. Political violence escalated in the late 1970s and into the 1980s and the victims were brought to Baragwanath. By the end of the 1980s, between 60 and 70 per cent of the surgical patient load was admitted as a result of some kind of trauma.[24]

Trauma victims arrived at surgical admissions, disparagingly known as the 'surgical pit'. This was a place of horrific human suffering, and its lack of resources meant that patients could die while waiting to be seen by a doctor or waiting for a bed; yet it also gave doctors the chance to practise and learn new techniques.[25] Developments included a new form of conservative therapy for parotid injury and innovative assessment management of head wounds, penetrating neck wounds and wounds to the abdomen which were seen in abundance at Baragwanath.[26] In a 1980s article dealing with arteriovenous fistulas and false aneurysms which occur after trauma, doctors wrote that the experience they gained from dealing with these cases at Baragwanath was 'usually only seen in war-time'.[27] Many of these developments were outlined in the 1988 publication *Modern Surgery in Africa: The Baragwanath Perspective*. It was said to be 'an important book for all doctors who work in Africa and has many messages for surgeons throughout the world ... For decades Baragwanath Hospital has held a reputation for unusual surgical pathology and its impressive trauma turnover and here is a book which describes an experience unique in the world.'[28] Similarly, Roger Saadia describes how the management strategy for hypovolaemic shock in patients with penetrating trauma was originally designed to relieve pressure on the busy resuscitation room by completing resuscitation and fluid replacement of the patient only on the operating table. It was found that this procedure had advantages in achieving haemodynamic stability. As Saadia noted; 'This is but one example where a management modality, born of necessity at Baragwanath Hospital, is found to have an intrinsic value in much better equipped trauma centres.'[29]

Experience such as this enabled Baragwanath's doctors to compete on the international stage. Years later, Chris van den Heever animates this point with a story:

In surgery, Mr Archie Stein published a huge series on the handling of various types of injuries, stab wounds to the chest, stab wounds of the abdomen, stab wounds of the neck, not a hundred cases but three or four or five thousand cases with various types of approaches. So you could imagine, when Archie stood up at a surgical meeting people listened, and not just local but overseas people too. I mean if you take the one example, they reported in the *Scandinavian Medical Journal* a stab wound of the chest sustained by a sailor and how everyone went 'gaga' about this and how everything that could go wrong with that patient did. When we saw that article here, Archie wrote to them and said, 'Look, this is what our experience is – whatever you did, do not do it again!' Then I was at a surgical congress here in Johannesburg where an American, an invited guest presented 300 stab wounds from Chicago, and when this was completed Professor du Plessis asked if Archie Stein was in the audience and he was. He was sitting right at the back and Du Plessis said Mr Stein would you like to comment and Archie got up and he said 'I don't agree with you' and sat down and Du Plessis asked how big Stein's series is on stabbed chests and he said, 'Oh about 4 500 cases,' and this American said, 'I'm sorry, I'm batting in the wrong league!'

The importance of these often-repeated stories in affirming the Baragwanath doctors should not be underestimated. The stories focused either on the expertise of the Baragwanath doctors and how this put them in a league of their own, or on the way in which international doctors came to gain experience and learn from the Baragwanath staff. Speaking in 2004, Max Price emphasised:

Everyone wants to feel that they are doing what the best in their profession can or are doing. As academics they go to international conferences and meet colleagues and it is important that they should not always feel that they are second rate and that people overseas are doing things that they can't hope to do because of resources or skills or technology. I think that is very important in keeping them here and in academia.

During the 1970s and 1980s a number of Baragwanath doctors took international fellowship exams for places such as Edinburgh, Dublin, London and Australia. Doctors suggested that there were two main motivations for this: taking the exams stood doctors who were unsure of their future in good stead should they wish to emigrate and at the same time, taking these exams could also have been part of a strategy for proving that they were equal to those who worked in these centres of medicine.[30] In an academic environment such as Baragwanath, gaining international recognition through such exams was encouraged.

Baragwanth also remained connected to the international medical community through its association with foreign doctors. Throughout the apartheid period, foreign doctors continued to come to Baragwanath despite boycotts and isolation. Many chose to come because of Baragwanath's reputation as a place where one could gain exceptionally varied clinical experience very quickly. For foreign doctors, clinical opportunities and exotic medical experiences were key appeals of Baragwanath but they were not the only draws. There were also foreign doctors who, like their local counterparts, found that Baragwanath fitted their social conscience and political motivations.

Foreign and local doctors both expressed the idea that the environment created at Baragwanath was one that allowed them to achieve a great deal as individuals in a milieu where one was often left to one's own devices. But at the same time many doctors reminiscing about their experiences emphasised the remarkable teamwork they found at Baragwanath. At a private or non-teaching hospital, a patient is cared for by a series of individual doctors. At teaching hospitals such as Baragwanath, one or two consultants, a handful of registrars, some interns and students all examine the patient and have to justify their decisions in a built-in, on the spot, participatory peer review process. This process should have led to the closer supervision of patients at Baragwanath but, according to David Seftel, the realities of a huge hospital, the workload and the tiered nature of the chain of command meant that the medical hierarchy often collapsed in the daily functioning of the hospital. Very little malpractice litigation, which could have led to tighter controls, occurred. One doctor said: 'you hoped you were doing the right thing and if you did not do the right thing then there was very little reprimand'. This meant that individual doctors often took on a great deal of individual responsibility.

Individuals were also able to champion projects and develop new areas of clinical practice and interest. Robert Lipschitz began to develop neurosurgery in the 1950s.[31] Lucy Wagstaff and PJ (Koos) Beukes championed the primary health clinics staffed by specially trained nurse-practitioners in the mid-1970s. Under the leadership of Issy Segal, the Gastroenterology Unit came into being in 1975; over the next decade it became one of the most important units of its kind in Africa, performing over 2 000 procedures annually and producing over 200 research contributions.[32] While patients benefited from these examples, this type of individualism raised concerns that the interests and egos of doctors could be put above the needs of patients in championing certain projects. This contradiction also highlights one of the central themes of this book: the availability of specialised medical care in the face of the lack of so many basic resources.

Many doctors point to the empowering freedom they felt they had at Baragwanath as an important aspect of their being there. Haroon Saloojee later explained:

> One of the things I have always said about Baragwanath, one person can make a huge difference at a place like Baragwanath. That is why I would never work in a place elsewhere overseas. There you are one cog in the wheel, at Baragwanath you are one and the power of one is essential.

For some doctors the sense of individual achievement was demonstrated in the heroic image they painted of themselves and their role at the hospital. This image is much more prevalent in written texts than oral interviews. Isadore Frack's description of his time as superintendent is filled with descriptions of crises which he almost singlehandedly solved, the one exception being his handling of the victims of the Sharpeville massacre which will be discussed later in this chapter.[33] Another doctor who gave a heroic autobiographic portrayal was surgeon John Hunt who worked at Baragwanath from 1964 until the late 1970s when he emigrated to the United States. The opening scene of Hunt's book describes how – dressed in a white coat and without gloves, which he did not have time to put on – he slashed open a patient's chest to do the internal heart compressions which returned the man from the dead.[34] He comments that 'what I had just now seen and done was beyond the bounds of ordinary human imagination. Even for surgeons.' This statement epitomises the way Hunt focused on the exotic, bizarre and sensational, and how he positioned himself in the 'doctor as hero' mould. In different ways, Hunt's and Frack's narratives both point to the importance that some doctors placed on the individual opportunities the hospital was perceived as affording them.

Individual responsibility was important, yet doctors also seemed to feel that they were expected to be part of the Baragwanath team. Several stressed teamwork and the cooperative spirit. As André Giraud said in 2004, it was 'busy and hard work but the spirit was phenomenal, there was a tremendous bond between people.' Ken Huddle concurred: 'There is a special camaraderie here which I have not found at other institutions. People work here because most of them are committed to helping rather poor and disadvantaged patients and that is a sort of bond that keeps people together. There are some exceptions but the majority of people are like that.' Others, like André Giraud, stressed teamwork in the face of a crisis:

> I remember many, many traumatic days at Bara when there were disasters, train accidents, or a fire that spread through the shacks – and suddenly there are three to four dozen or 200 patients! And now let me tell you the moment that happens, if I was on intake when I got busy, all of a sudden all the other units came to help, even the gynaecologists and paediatricians! And they examine and help even if it has nothing to do with them. The gynaecologists would come for a train accident – they would clerk the patients.

Apart from the train accidents, fires and natural disasters, the political turmoil of the country also led to moments of crisis. On 21 March 1960, Baragwanath's superintendent got word that the Vereeniging Hospital was ill-equipped to deal with the large number of serious gunshot cases in the aftermath of the Sharpeville massacre and that the patients would be transferred to Baragwanath. 'Operation disaster' was put in place, wards were emptied of all patients who could be sent home and emergency equipment was prepared. Frack stressed that 'everyone knew his or her job and I was a proud man that day'. Teamwork allowed the hospital to cope with sixty-nine dead and 143 wounded and to perform 66 major operations in under twenty-four hours. Surgeons, anaesthetists and theatre nurses from various units acted in relays.[35] In the aftermath of the shooting, Frack was placed on compulsory leave for no apparent reason. Suggestions have been made that he embarrassed the government by stressing in a press conference that the victims were shot in the back. After threats that many of the staff would leave the hospital with him, Frack was reinstated.[36]

On 16 June 1976 it was again Baragwanath that treated victims of political violence. At Sharpeville the massacre happened far from the hospital, but in 1976 Baragwanath was right in the heart of the violence. It was not a single shooting with a defined number of patients. Victims of political violence continued to flow into the hospital for months after the initial uprising. The proximity of the violence affected members of the hospital's staff who worried about their own safety. Yet, it was also a crisis that saw people pull together. One doctor remembers: 'On 16 June 1976 I was on intake – I will never forget it, we all worked through the night, it does not matter, not only my unit but the other units helping.'[37] There was also pride in the fact that Baragwanath was self-sufficient: 'Help had been offered to Baragwanath by other hospitals on the Reef but had been refused.'[38] Doctors' discussions of the response of the staff to the uprisings are also significant in that it was the only time during my interviews that doctors seemed to point to a racial divide between nurses and doctors. They remembered the tension that built up between themselves and nurses who refused to help treat black policemen or those they saw as collaborators. Other doctors remembered being threatened and even spat upon.[39]

It was, in the eyes of many doctors, a tremendous team effort that allowed Baragwanath to cope in these situations. The ideas about teamwork were also emphasised as significant in order to show that the staff at Baragwanath were self-sufficient within their specific teams. This was important when they were isolated both physically and socially from what were generally considered the centres of medical power.

Politics, humanitarianism and institutional commitment

Baragwanath Hospital was a place that corresponded with many doctors' political and social identities. Reg Broekman, a doctor and long time hospital administrator, later commented in an interview: 'I think a lot of the senior clinicians are there for ethical reasons, they believe they have a commitment to help serve the public sector.' These objectives, whether rooted in a humanitarian philosophy, in religious motivations or in political activism, led doctors to feel that they had a role to play at Baragwanath.

I think it became clear to me that my home would always be Baragwanath. I think it is clear why it is … particularly in paediatrics, and also the other areas I have been in. Baragwanath was the area most in need. So it was fulfilling the need to serve people most in need. I think it offered a home that I was comfortable with.

This need to help people, as expressed by Haroon Saloojee, a politically active and socially conscious doctor of Indian descent, was, unsurprisingly, a common theme in doctors' stated motivations for going into medicine, both in oral material and in their non-clinical writing. David Blumsohn, a less politically active but equally social conscious doctor, expressed a common philosophy and motivation among doctors at Baragwanath and more generally when he states that he aimed 'to always be a good doctor, be a good human being and to help people'. From the time he started participating in teaching rounds at Baragwanath as a student in the mid 1950s, Blumsohn – who was often referred to as 'the conscience of Baragwanath' by his colleagues – felt that the hospital gave scope to develop these motives.[40] Even as a student he and some of his peers went, by his own account, beyond the call of duty: 'we used to come out even at times we did not have to and help with ward rounds and we saw patients, it seemed to me to be the ideal way to practice medicine'. People such as Blumsohn present the hospital as a place where people worked because they felt morally bound by a love for humanity. For many doctors this idea manifests in the fight for better conditions for their patients in the hope that 'one day someone somewhere will believe the truth for what it is that our patients deserve better'. Ken Huddle, who also seems to have been driven by a sense of social and moral consciousness, expands on the idea of the doctor as patient advocate. He notes that Baragwanath's patients 'have been downtrodden and browbeaten for so long that we took on the role of complaining and doing the protesting... and we have had a lot of protests for our patients over the years which we have not seen at other institutions.' Many Baragwanath doctors suggested that although they worked in an incredibly difficult environment, it was one in which they could help those who were less fortunate than themselves and be a voice for them. This particular hospital was one for which they felt that they had a moral and ethical responsibility that went above medicine alone.[41]

Despite apartheid laws making separate kitchens, toilets, living facilities and lounges compulsory, the hospital was a fairly multiracial space in its daily functioning. Although there were the hierarchies that one would find in any hospital setting – senior over junior, doctor over nurse and, in the South African setting, white over black – these patterns were sometimes complicated by daily interactions. The nature of medical work in the wards meant that white doctors worked side by side with black doctors and nurses on a daily basis. Desmond Pantanowitz described his experience of racial mixing at Baragwanath during the 1980s as follows:

> It was after all the days of apartheid, and social mixing was frowned upon by the government. But it did happen at Bara. I think most of the doctors and nurses got on very well and I think it was the medical profession that demonstrated that people of different races could get on well, and they did. From my perspective people got on very well and in contrast to the whole apartheid philosophy Bara showed that you could, that the races could, get on very well and there was good intersocial contact at Bara.

Several doctors echoed Pantanowitz's view that Baragwanath was a place of social racial mixing. For others there was a silence around issues of race, despite the pervasiveness of racial issues in South Africa. One strand of thinking among a particular segment of Baragwanath doctors was that 'you don't talk politics and religion; this is a place of the sick'. André Giraud, a French Mauritian who did his medical training at Wits during the 1950s and spent three decades at Baragwanath, commented that '[politics] did not seem to affect us – you know, we heard what was going on, but everybody was in the same boat. It did not affect the running of the hospital at all; these racial implications were not there.' Many doctors and nurses commented on the good working relationships between the two professional groups at Baragwanath hospital. Their overwhelmingly positive response to each other could have been influenced by the fact that they were talking to me as a young white woman, but it seemed that the nature of these relationships was an important aspect of the way nurses and doctors spoke about their experiences at Baragwanath. These relationships were not always straightforward. A number of doctors explained how it was often the matron who could wield power in the wards, and from the 1960s matrons at Baragwanath were increasingly African women. In an interview, David Seftel explains his perception of this relationship during the late 1970s and into the 1980s:

> This was a time when grand apartheid was still very much in force, PW Botha was putting new rules in place and nobody knew that liberation

was really coming. There was definitely a hierarchy in the nursing profession that shaped attitudes. To a young doctor this could be quite severe. You feared the matron more than you feared your supervising doctor in many cases, because the matron had the power to make your life as an intern's life hell. They are the people who would call you at 2 am, 3 am and 4 am if they did not like you; they are the ones who would refuse to do things that you might ask them to do or to tell their nurses not to take instructions from you. There was a lot of this subtle power struggle ... it was a kind of hierarchical rivalry ... because I think traditionally the one area in which nurses had more power was as matrons and they had more power than the doctors and at Bara this was one area in which they could wield their authority and they did.

A black doctor, Haroon Saloojee gave a view of race relations which was more complicated:

For a lot of my period, the 80s ... my sense of Bara is unfortunately linked partially to a racial issue. We had a black identity at Bara and obviously by black I mean, Indian, coloured and African ... We had our own teas, we had a certain culture, we had a friendship and that persisted and that unfortunately did define the Baragwanath experience for me in the early years.

Yet he went on to say that race did not have a significant effect on the quality of care:

Fortunately, I don't think that ever became a race issue. I don't think I would seriously argue that my white colleagues were necessarily, I am talking in the Bara environment, behaving in ways that were severely less ethical than my black colleagues. I think that tended to transcend the racial issue, there were bad black doctors and there were bad white doctors.

Thus, while the hospital could be seen as a contested multiracial space, the hospital itself was, according to Haroon Saloojee, 'situated in a particular site that was a hotbed of change in the country and people at the institution were often prominent people in other political activities'. Political activists, especially those among the white doctors, felt that at Baragwanath they were surrounded by like-minded people and it was a place from where they could be involved in the broader struggle. Baragwanath Hospital offered a space in which their identity as white doctors was formed, not as part of the apartheid regime, but by being able to work against the regime from within a state institution. There are also examples of the hospital offering a multiracial space in which politically active doctors could organise and educate.

It was at Baragwanath that Dr Neil Aggett became involved in championing workers' rights through his work as an organiser with the Transvaal Food and Canning Workers' Union. The popular doctor, who learned isiZulu in an attempt to understand and communicate with his patients, was instrumental in organising the successful Fattis and Monis strike in Isando in 1979 as well as other mass action campaigns. In late 1981, Neil Aggett was detained. He died in detention on 5 February 1982 at the age of twenty-nine. The official cause of death was suicide by hanging. A later inquest revealed that his death was as a result of police torture. He became the first white person to die in detention since 1963 and was the fifty-first person to die in this way.

Among the Baragwanath community stories abound about activists either on the staff, as patients, or moving through the hospital as 'visitors' handing out literature, putting up political posters or organising meetings.[42] There were also stories of individual doctors harbouring struggle patients. David Seftel explained how the responsibility bestowed on individuals, although terrifying, allowed him to protect political detainees:

In a circumstance where I was treating detainees I was in a position where I could say 'I am not letting this patient be discharged', and as long as I documented on the patient's chart that there were medical reasons for doing so I was unable to be overturned ... I could keep them until they were strong enough ... That is not to say that at certain points in time, Van Den Heever (the superintendent) would be called by the military and they would say 'we have a problem with some stupid doctors who do not want to discharge our patients'. At that point I got questioned and my response to that was to say – using the chart – that the person could not be discharged.

It is not surprising that Baragwanath attracted doctors whose professional motivations were intertwined with their politics and who were driven to medicine by the same sense of social action that led them into activism. Numerous early black doctors were involved in political organisations. Dilizantaba Mji, who did his internship at Baragwanath, was head of the Transvaal Youth League and an African National Congress (ANC) executive member.[43] There were several white doctors who were politically active. Some of them portrayed their political involvement in terms of broader social action. Max Price, for example, saw medicine as 'one profession that had more of a social impact than others'. For David Seftel, who grew up in a medical and activist family and whose parents had been doctors at Baragwanath for many years, 'public service and activism were closely linked'.

Among the early activists were South African born doctors Effie Shultz (David Seftel's mother) and Yahuda Kaplan. Shultz, one of a handful of women doctors working at the hospital during the 1950s, was actively involved in the struggle for equal pay for doctors of different races and in the protests against the introduction of the new Nursing Act in 1957 which will be discussed in Chapter 5. Shultz was reluctant to speak about her role in these events but she was often mentioned in political circles. When asked in an interview about fellow activists at Baragwanath in the 1950s, Yahuda Kaplan asked, 'Have you heard of Effie Shultz? She was a lot more left wing and active than I was.' Another doctor who was at Baragwanath at the time, recalled:

> Effie had a room next to mine at Bara when we were housemen, and she said to me one morning my room is a bit small and could I keep her books, so she put them under my bed and it was all her communist literature – under my bed, she was concerned that there would be problems but thought they would not suspect me.

Yahuda Kaplan began working at Baragwanath in 1956. He became the first person to be fired from the hospital for political action – or, as the hospital administration put it, for 'mixing with non-whites'. Unlike many politicised doctors Kaplan did not have a political upbringing. He explains that he 'was blinkered like the rest of white South Africans until I became a medical student. There were coloured and Indian students in my class, and I can't remember if we had any black South Africans in medicine, that was when my eyes were opened, so to speak.' However, it was not activism that led Kaplan, who had trained at the University of Cape Town, to Baragwanath.

I fell madly in love with a nurse doing maternity and midwifery training and I knew she was going back to work at Bara. So I thought that I wanted to go too ... Well it was the main reason. My cousin was married to one of the consultant ENT surgeons at Bara and he managed to get me a post as a senior houseman and that was how I got to Bara.

When he and the Muslim nurse arrived at Baragwanath they found that the staff members were separated into different residences based on race and that social integration between the races was frowned upon. Outraged, Kaplan looked for a means to express his discontent. He did this by joining the Congress Movement.[44] It was at one of these meetings that he met the woman he was later to marry, a young but prominent anti-apartheid lawyer. The two continued political work from their rooms in the hospital's white doctors' quarters:

> We did not have any qualms about inviting black doctors or nurses into our rooms and we also took classes with groups of medical orderlies and taught them trade unionism and socialism. We used to ferry some of them back to Soweto at night afterwards. I was also selling the Congress Newspaper ... and that is what got me kicked out.[45]

Baragwanath became part of Kaplan's political awakening and the centre for his activism. He talks about Baragwanath as a special place where it was possible to learn about medicine and politics. He summed up his feelings by saying: 'I would have spent the rest of my life at Bara, if I had not been kicked out, that was my intention'. Like Kaplan's, Effie Shultz's career at Baragwanath was cut short when she applied for a senior houseman's post. The TPA refused to authorise her for the position because of her engagement in political activity.[46]

By the 1970s the make-up of doctors at Baragwanath began to change. During the early years of that decade a number of politically active doctors had resigned or been fired. At the same time, as Helen Rees explained, 'Among politically active people it was not at all encouraged to go into management, so very, very few people went into that.' When politically active people worked their way up the system to a point where they would be promoted into management, many left the public health care system. After the Soweto uprisings later in the decade, some doctors fled Soweto and Baragwanath.

Nevertheless, a new group of young, politicised doctors replaced them in the post-1976 period and directly confronted the conditions in which black South Africans lived. Max Price pointed out that:

> Medical students in the late 70s ... were highly politicised and much more so than any other faculty of students ... I think they were so politicised because of their exposure to a part of society that most whites never saw. Besides that they were going into Soweto almost every day to go to Bara and so there was the panorama of Soweto and life there. There was the contact with patients. There was the obvious consequence of malnutrition, of poverty, infectious disease, STDs, TB, trauma and alcoholism. In addition, we were there when the riots took place so we would be in casualty and we would have dozens of kids coming in peppered with gun shots and you would see patients in bed with police there guarding them and people brought in from prison. And so I think white students, white medical students confronted much more directly than almost any other students what was going on ... I think Bara was very politicising for white students.

Some doctors, black and white, and many nurses, were politicised by what they saw, but this was certainly not universal. I have already mentioned those who had very little contact with the community outside the hospital and on the other hand there were doctors, including Price, who were politically active long before they set foot in medical school.

Price came from a medical family and at school had been involved in mobilising white youth to demonstrate against apartheid human rights abuses such as the murder of Ahmed Timol.[47] During his time as an intern at Baragwanath, he continued to lead such protests. For example, he coordinated a petition calling for doctors to resign from the Medical Association of South Africa over the 'Biko Doctors' Affair.[48] Price was influential, and others I interviewed stressed this. Chris van den Heever said:

> In 1980, my first full year here, we had a group of students including Max Price ... they certainly made a huge impact on the student community and you know the sort of person you are dealing with, Price was very eloquent, very persuasive, always balanced – but you

knew what you were dealing with – you were dealing with a very sharp opponent.

Another doctor who came to Baragwanath already politicised was Haroon Saloojee. During his school years in the 1970s he travelled 30 kilometres to school in Lenasia each day because as an Indian he was prohibited from attending one of the white schools situated around his home in the city. He says:

> I remember very well the 1976 riots ... In subsequent days clearly we were meeting all our African counterparts as we went by Soweto in the train. We shared our *amandlas*. But clearly at school level already I got into trouble because there were solidarity meetings with the Soweto students. So, yeah, the activism was not necessarily related to medicine it is just that now that I am in medicine that continues of course.

During the 1980s and 1990s he continued broader political work as well as fighting for the Baragwanath patients in campaigns such as 'Save Our Babies', and later through work with the Treatment Action Campaign (TAC) to make HIV/AIDS drugs available through the public health care system.

As this group of doctors was entering the system, the head of the Department of Medicine changed. Vernon Wilson retired in the early 1970s and Leo Schamroth took over as head. He was a tireless campaigner for patients' rights and, while his focus was within the hospital, he created an environment in which those involved in broader political struggles felt comfortable. Some activists actually saw Baragwanath as a safe haven although this was never uncontested. Kaplan originally saw Baragwanath as a place he could organise and educate during the 1950s, yet the hospital proved to be anything but a safe place for him. Others saw the main change as coming later. David Seftel suggested that 'for a while it was a safe haven, but then the spies infiltrated in the 1980s'. The extent to which this is true is hard to ascertain. There were certainly many rumours and stories about spies infiltrating the hospital and some doctors mentioned this during interviews. However, a decade later Saloojee felt that:

> From a personal perspective Baragwanath was useful for me as a safe haven. Because of political involvement I had, at various stages, held

offices in various parts of what was called the Johannesburg Youth Congress and we would regularly have members picked up by the security police. I remember a time when I was treasurer, what I would do is use Bara as my safe house. I had my own cupboard in the Paeds ward and so I kept my things there.

However, Saloojee also added a word of caution by talking about the police roadblocks often placed on the road to Baragwanath.

At Baragwanath, a hospital staffed predominantly by white doctors treating black patients in the apartheid era, race played out in complex ways. To some extent the attitude of some white doctors could be compared to those of missionaries or humanitarians. Chris van den Heever commented that people outside the hospital saw those who worked there as 'missionaries'. Mission hospitals, however, were often part of a 'civilising' or 'westernising' process, and members of the medical staff at Baragwanath were not explicitly aiming to 'civilise' Soweto. Thus Van den Heever may have used the word 'missionary' in order to highlight the humanitarian nature of the work.

There were a few who represented their motives for serving at Baragwanath in religious terms. Anaesthesiologist and long-time Baragwanath doctor George Veliotes joked that '[t]hose of us who have been here for a long time say you either have to be mad, bad or religious to stay at Baragwanath'.[49] Among the most well-known religious people linked to the hospital in the early years were the Rev. EH Sobukwe – brother of the African intellectual and Pan Africanist Congress founder Robert Sobukwe – and the Rev. Martin Jarrett-Kerr. Jarrett-Kerr, of the Community of the Resurrection in the United Kingdom, ministered for seven years at the only church on the hospital premises, the Chapel of St Luke, built by the Anglicans during the war. Others, such as Rev. Dr Liz Carmichael, had the dual role of ministering to patients and providing medical care. Carmichael, who was a candidate with one of the major Church of England missionary societies, describes how her coming to work in South Africa was influenced by meeting, during a brief trip in 1972, people like Beyers Naude, Helen Joseph and the nuns of the Little Sisters of Jesus, who were trying to create a different life for those in their order and those among whom they worked under apartheid. She returned to South Africa in 1975 and worked as a doctor at Baragwanath until 1981.[50] Over a decade earlier, Peggie Preston, a British occupational therapist, had also felt driven to come to South Africa and seek work at Baragwanath after being influenced by Alan Paton's book *Cry the Beloved Country* and by her Anglican beliefs. Both women seem to have come to South Africa out of an interest in the country itself rather than Baragwanath; however, once in the country they suggest that the hospital complemented the kind of work they wanted to do and the people they wished to serve. As foreigners and with a religious base, both were able to engage with the community around them. Preston spoke fondly about her escapades around Soweto with her friend Iris, a Baragwanath nurse and singer, and the especially colourful nights at Dorkay House, a multiracial music and performance space in Eloff Street, central Johannesburg, frequented by artists and intellectuals. Similarly, Carmichael pointed out that her situation was:

> ... slightly different from that of all of my colleagues, in that I really knew people in Soweto. As a Brit, coming from outside, I had no qualms about it and in fact I was keen to get into Soweto and get to know people ... It was through church contacts that I got to know a whole lot of people around my own age, that was 20s, particularly in Diepkoof. A club spontaneously formed – it was called the Diepkloof Progress Cultural Club. It had about 30 members and we did all the things we could do together. We went to Zoo Lake, we hired boats, because it was Lions Club and we could do that together. We went to Sterkfontein Caves because that belonged to Wits and we could do that.

Over and above her work at Baragwanath, Carmichael played an active role as convenor of the Alexandra Interim Crisis Committee and was involved in the National Peace Accord in the early 1990s.

The personal religious beliefs of several other doctors guided them to 'do good' in their individual lives and thus at the hospital. Reg Broekman described religion as one of the factors that led doctors to do good work. Beukes believes that being brought up in a religious tradition taught him the values he needed to be superintendent of Baragwanath hospital between 1974 and 1980. In his unpublished autobiography he writes:

> I was raised in the tradition, or shall I say, brought up in the culture of hard work, taking responsibility, honesty, religiousness, respect for others, independence, self-reliance, self-supporting, dexterity,

integrity, altruism, setting an example, to consider every obstacle as a challenge – a stepping stone to achieve success.[51]

In this statement, as indeed in the book as a whole, Beukes shows that he is clearly driven by the Afrikaner values of a pious devotion to God, hard work and a deep respect for stoicism. Writing 27 years after the events he recorded, when he was in his eighties, he devoted a great deal of space to an explanation of how these values were formed during his unsettled youth spent trekking in an ox-wagon from farm to farm in Namaqualand. Throughout the text, he stressed that these values led him to succeed in medicine and at Baragwanath during one of its most difficult periods. He was a quintessential 'Bara Boetie'.

While religion was a guiding force for some doctors, it played almost no role in the self-presentation of most of those I interviewed. There were several Jewish doctors at Baragwanath throughout the period I researched. Jarrett-Karr, writing in the 1960s about his experiences during the previous decade, noted that: 'at our own hospital [Baragwantath] we have a preponderance of Jewish doctors'.[52] I interviewed quite a few Jewish doctors, but their Jewish identity hardly came to the fore. Despite this, they were grouped together by others. For example, Peggy Preston, commenting on her experiences in the early 1960s said: 'What I saw at that time was that the people who were really helping the Africans mostly were the Jews'. Chris van den Heever also referred to the Jewish doctors at Baragwanath. 'You had the guys from St Johns's College at Jo'burg Hospital, and those from King David at Bara'.[53] David Seftel was the only Jewish doctor I interviewed to comment on this topic. He said, 'It is just so fascinating, if you look at the cast of characters in this play – they were probably some of the most prominent members of the Jewish community in this country. On one side you have activists and on the other side you have collaborators. This was discussed, but not brought to the fore.' While religion and culture might have had an influence on Jewish doctors' decisions to go into medicine, or on the way they practised their profession, it was difficult to discern this from the interviews.

Bara Boeties

In contrast to the political focus of some of Baragwanath's doctors, there were those whose commitment to the hospital existed in relative isolation from broader social and political struggles. According to Chris van den Heever they were 'dedicated to the hospital and could see the good and the bad but would fight to improve it'. It was their lack of involvement in the broader political struggles that seems to have motivated David Seftel to comment that 'those who called themselves "Bara Boeties" only looked internally'. A number of doctors, including Seftel, expressed a sceptical view of the 'Bara Boeties' in interviews and in general conversations because of their uncertain political leanings and because the concept was often linked to hospital administrators. Indeed, Beukes, who served as chief superintendent during the 1970s, and his successor Van den Heever, self-identified, and were identified by others, as Bara Boeties. It was during their tenures that the term gained prominence. This was also a time when working conditions were becoming increasingly arduous. Against this background, the term seems to have emerged as a way of pointing to and reinforcing the qualities doctors saw as important at Baragwanath.

Chris van den Heever had first come to Baragwanath as a Wits student during the early 1960s. He graduated in 1965 and became an intern at Baragwanath in 1966. He then worked at South Rand Hospital until 1976, when he came to Baragwanath as deputy superintendent. In 1980 he took over the reins as chief superintendent, a position he held until 1999. Although officially in retirement, he was often at the hospital during the period from 2003 to 2005 when I visited the hospital regularly, and he continued to serve the hospital in an advisory capacity. This type of long-term involvement and commitment was seen as an important marker of a 'Bara Boetie'. Van den Heever's pride in the hospital and his desire to preserve its place in history were evident in his passion for the hospital's history. He wrote articles and collected a vast amount of historical material, to much of which I had access.

Commitment was important. André Giraud said:

From 1962 to 1980 I was at Bara. It was not the first time I came to Bara, I did the senior house job at Baragwanath in obstetrics and gynaecology in 1953. Then I was away, while others stayed here for long time. Here you found that when you were away and came back you had to be tested and then OK.

The idea of commitment being 'tested' before full acceptance seems to have been very much part of the Baragwanath culture. It was something that was also pointed out by nurses, as will be discussed in the next chapter. It suggests that certain doctors and nurses saw a collective Baragwanath identity to which one could belong if one was seen as having the characteristics of a Bara Boetie.

Being a Bara Botie was not only about the length of time one spent at Baragwanath, although that was clearly important. Giraud felt that others interpreted his having left the hospital and then returned as demonstrating his lack of commitment – however, he was able to prove his loyalty to the hospital in other ways. One important aspect of the Bara Boeties was their pride in the hospital and what it could do. Some spoke with such confidence about the hospital that they said they would want to be treated there. André Giraud explained that he would ' ... often tell my wife if ever I have a medical problem I know where I want to be treated – I want to go to Baragwanath'. It was commitment to the hospital that led Van den Heever to end his farewell speech to Anna Marie Richter, one of the assistant superintendents during the 1980s, by saying that her commitment to, pride in and work at the hospital meant that she was 'en sal jy 'n Bara Boetie bly'.[54]

Koos Beukes did not have a long history at the hospital. He was born in 1924 on a farm near Springbok in Namaqualand and his worldview was shaped by the Afrikaner values of his youth. He also credits his upbringing with providing him the strength of character and respect for people of all races that he needed to run a hospital such as Baragwanath. He wrote that it was Feitjie, the daughter of the African women who worked in his family's kitchen and with whom he played as a child, who taught him to value people of all races.[55] After studying at the Universities of Stellenbosch and Pretoria where he specialised in surgery, he worked for the provincial administration, mining corporations and in private practice before being asked to join the staff at Baragwanath as deputy superintendent in the early 1970s. After just eight months he was promoted to superintendent at South Rand Hospital. However, his stay there was equally brief and he was transferred back to Baragwanath. He spent only six years at the helm of the hospital before stepping down to the post of deputy superintendent in 1980 owing to ill health.

Beukes is a contradictory person. On one hand he trained at conservative Afrikaans universities and worked for the TPA and the mining industry, yet during his time at Baragwanath he came across as liberal in all his dealings with others. Black nurses, many of whom had worked with him in the primary health clinics during the 1980s, seemed to have a genuine warmth and respect for him; many call him *Oom Koos*, Uncle Koos. People of all races seemed to respect his pride in the hospital and his commitment to its ideals. One white doctor commented, 'I remember him particularly well ... I particularly liked him. He was a Bara Boetie for sure. He did a lot for the hospital and was very understanding, he made sure it was clean and made sure it was well stocked and had good doctors. Beukes was someone very special.' In speeches and newspaper articles celebrating his retirement in 1989, a number of people commented on his total devotion to the hospital and to his job. Beukes explains his own contribution to Baragwanath as follows:

> In my own opinion I made a considerable contribution towards the sick, disadvantaged and poor people in my own community and I had felt that it was my duty and obligation to do the same towards other societies and races. I saw Baragwanath Hospital as the stepping stone to eventually reach my goal. That was probably why I enjoyed my work at Baragwanath Hospital so much.[56]

The term 'Bara Boetie' also seemed to have been used by the administration to present the image of the ideal Baragwanath doctor. The section of the 'Barameter' (the bi-annual staff newsletter introduced during the 1980s) which dealt with staff promotions, awards and retirements was headed 'Bara Boetie'. Black and white staff appeared together on these pages. A cartoon, which appeared in the same publication, featured the exploits of a character named 'Bara Boetie'.

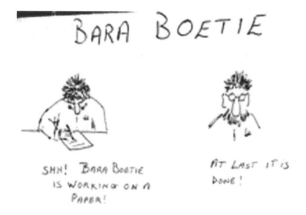

Figure 2: Excerpt from 'Bara Boetie Cartoon'[57]

Among the doctors said to be Bara Boeties it was Van den Heever and Beukes who epitomised the concept by their way of thinking and talking about the hospital and their pride in its development and clinical excellence. They believed in the positive image of the hospital that they portrayed. Yet they also perpetuated a façade which masked many of the underlying difficulties that the hospital faced. I will return to this theme in Chapter 6.

The Baragwanath doctors

Many of the Baragwanath doctors spoke about how fulfilling and rewarding their experiences were, on both personal and professional levels. While not all would self-identify, or would be identified, as Bara Boeties, they share fundamental elements of identity. Their motivations, sphere of influence and working identity were rooted within the hospital and the unique and specific experience it offered on a number of levels. Many doctors who worked at Baragwanath spoke about it in positive, sometimes even glowing terms – even while acknowledging its difficulties and problems. However, the context of apartheid was ever-present in the hospital and had a significant effect on the experiences of both black and white doctors and on patient care. In trying to understand the doctors' motivations and ways of presenting the hospital, the issue of how these factors translated into patient care or, indeed, whether notions of clinical excellence were real or perceived, is less important than the fact that these issues are important to the way in which the doctors see themselves and how they talk about their experiences at Baragwanath. In the face of difficult conditions the doctors rallied together around the one point they had in common – the hospital. In interviews and in their writing, they claimed insider knowledge of how good the hospital really was. Buddy Lawson, looking back on his career at Baragwanath, summed it up: 'Some uneducated people will look down on Bara but they don't know what is going on. If you are full-time and you take that seriously then it is a very fulfilling place'.

For the doctors who identified with the hospital the positive aspect of Baragwanath's image was vital. Their heroic descriptions of the hospital and their ability not only to cope with, but even to thrive in, the conditions there, was an important justification for being there and a validation of their skills in the face of often disparaging remarks by outsiders. Lucy Wagstaff, who joined the Paediatric Department at Baragwanath in 1964, hints at something important in this presentation of the hospital when she notes: 'Bara had a special global reputation for a very long time ... we had innovative ways of doing things. In many ways it is some kind of family thing, inside Bara people could know about the problems but if anyone came from outside it was different.'

Doctors, in their memoirs and recollections, in pamphlets, reports and in articles about the hospital often stressed the positive image of Baragwanath. Some doctors saw Baragwanath as a good place to be professionally for those who focused on clinical work and those whose focus was on medical research and publishing. The access to an unusually large patient load with a variety of chronic and acute ailments as well as close links to the Wits medical school meant that despite the frustrations and poor conditions at the hospital, Baragwanath offered an unrivalled experience to those who worked there. As a result, a number of clinicians and researchers whose work was widely recognised chose to stay at Baragwanath. This is perhaps counter-intuitive given the limits that the chronic over-crowding and understaffing imposed on doctors at the hospital.

For others, the humanitarian aspects of working among the poor and oppressed chimed with their personal philosophies. The hospital attracted some with primarily religious motivations. Others were more overtly political. Among these politically active doctors were those who held official positions within the liberation movements and who tended to see their work at the hospital as part of the broader struggle for the rights of the black population – and at the same time saw the ability to organise politically and to protect and treat victims of apartheid as advantages of working at Baragwanath. They were a diverse group who put different weights on these professional, personal or political ideologies, but many shared one thing in common – the view that the hospital was distinctive. A select group among them were identified by themselves and others as 'Bara Boeties'and were said to embody the spirit of Baragwanath Hospital.[58]

Endnotes

1   See also 'Baragwanath "Snubbed" Doctors Say Few Wits Medical Students Visit the Hospital', *Sunday Times*, 24 March 1964.

2   WHF Kenny (1969) 'Baragwanath Hospital's Twenty-First Birthday'. *South African Medical Journal*, 43:21, May, p. 601.

3   DMF, L Schamroth, response to the Claude Harris Leon Foundation Award, 9 March 1985.

4   On diseases of the alimentary canal see KJ Keeley (1958) 'Alimentary Disease in the Bantu', *Medical Proceedings*, 4:10, May, pp. 281–6. On the relationship between traditional medicines and these diseases see H Grusin (1955) 'Potassium Dichromate as a Witchdoctor's Remedy; Five Cases of Poisoning'. *South African Medical Journal* 29:6, February, pp. 117–20. On scurvy at Baragwanath see H Grusin and PS Kincaid-Smith (1954) 'Scurvy in Adult Africans: A Clinical, Hematological, and Pathological Study'. *American Journal of Clinical Nutrition* 2:5, September–October, pp. 323–35.

5   H Stein and EU Rosen (1980) 'Changing Trends in Child Health in Soweto: The Baragwanath Hospital Picture'. *South African Medical Journal* 58:26, December, pp. 1 030–2.

6   Altmann (1948) op. cit., pp. 32–5; A Altmann and CG Anderson (1951) Electrophoretic Serum Protein Pattern in Malignant Malnutrition. *Lancet* 1:4, January.

7   CG Bremner (1971) 'The Changing Pattern of Disease seen at Baragwanath Hospital'. *South African Journal of Surgery* 9:3, July–September, pp. 127–31.

8   See for example I Segal and JA Hunt (1975) 'The Irritable Bowel Syndrome in the Urban South African Negro'. *South African Medical Journal* 49:40, September, pp. 1 645–6; I Segal, LO Tim, A Solomon and A Giraud (1978) 'Diverticular Disease in Urban Blacks'. *South African Medical Journal* 53:23, June, p. 922; and AR Walker and I Segal (1979) 'Is Appendicitis Increasing in South African Blacks?' *South African Medical Journal* 56:13, September, pp. 503–4.

9   AR Walker and I Segal (1979) 'Epidemiology of Noninfective Intestinal Diseases in Various Ethnic Groups in South Africa'. *Israel Journal of Medical Sciences* 15:4, April, pp. 309–13.

10 S Barold (1996) 'Leo Schamroth (1924–1988): His Life and Work'. *Journal of Medical Biographies*, 4:3, August, pp. 125–8. Among his most famous books are *The Disorders of Cardiac Rhythm* (Oxford, 1971) and *Electrocardiology*

of *Coronary Artery Disease* (Oxford, 1984). His last work, a four-volume tome, was published posthumously: *Twelve Lead Electrocardiography* (Oxford, 1989).

11 DMF, L Schamroth, Response to the Claude Harris Leon Foundation Award, 9 March 1985.

12 Frack (1958a) op. cit.

13 Moria Russell, in a letter to Simonne Horwitz, 6 April 2004.

14 W Edelstein (1971) 'The Management of Transverse Lie in Labour'. *South African Journal of Obstetrics and Gynaecology* 4, May, p. 18.

15 D Parekh and HH Lawson (1987) 'Gallstone Disease among Black South Africans: A Review of the Baragwanath Hospital Experience'. *South African Medical Journal* 72:1, July, p. 23.

16 André Giraud, 12 July 2004 and David Blumsohn, 27 September 2004 discussed this at some length.

17 I Segal and LO Tim (1979) 'The Witchdoctor and the Bowel'. *South African Medical Journal* 56:8, August, pp. 308–10. A similar argument for a later period can be found in D Pantanowitz (1995) *Alternative Medicine: A Doctor's Perspective.* Cape Town: Southern.

18 SR Benatar (1991) 'Medicine and Health Care in South Africa – Five Years Later'. *New England Journal of Medicine* 325:1, July, pp. 30–6 and A Seedat (1984) *Crippling a Nation: Health in Apartheid South Africa.* London: IDAF, p. 12.

19 Giraud RMA, I Luke and A Schmaman (1969) 'Crohn's Disease in the Transvaal Bantu: A Report of 5 Cases'. *South African Medical Journal* 43:21, May, pp. 610–2.

20 Eisenstein (1977) 'The Morphology and Pathological anatomy of Lumber Spine in South African Negro and Caucasoid with Specific Reference to Spinal Stenosis'. *Journal of Bone Joint Surgery* 59:2, May, pp. 173–88.

21 DV Meerkotter and J Craig (1988) 'Spinal Stenosis at Baragwanath Hospital, Johannesburg'. *South African Journal of Surgery,* 26:1, March, pp. 10–2.

22 R Saadia (1999) 'Organisation of Hospital Responses for the Trauma Epidemic'. *British Medical Bulletin* 55:4, p. 782.

23 C van den Heever (1991) 'Baragwanath, Africa's Largest Hospital'. *Africa Business and Chamber of Commerce Review* (Medical Supplement) 27:17, January, p. 37; Frack, *Every Man,* p. 193.

24 HH Lawson (1988) Preface, in D Pantanowitz (ed.) *Modern Surgery in Africa: The Baragwanath Experience.* Johannesburg: Southern, pp. 3–82;

I Segal (1988) 'The Trauma of the Urban Experience'. *Journal of the Royal College of Physicians London* 22:1, January, pp. 45–7. During oral interviews the changing types of trauma were discussed by Reg Broekman, 27 July 2004; Annah Ntshangase, 19 August 2004 and Mpe Tenza, 5 October 2004.

25 Hebestreit op. cit., pp. 672–3; Saadia op. cit., pp. 767–80.

26 See, for example D Pantanowitz (ed.) (1988) *Modern Surgery in Africa: The Baragwanath Experience.* Johannesburg: Southern, pp. 33, 39, 48 and S Kleinot (1958) 'The Work of the Surgical Division'. *Medical Proceedings* 4:10, May, pp. 286–92.

27 J Franklin and C Hatzitheofilou (1987) 'Arteriovenous Fistulas and False Aneurysms Occurring after Trauma'. *South African Journal of Surgery* 25:3, September, pp. 79–84.

28 CG Bremner (1998) 'Modern Surgery in Africa: The Baragwanath Experience: A Book Review'. *South African Journal of Science* 84:11, November, p. 923.

29 Saadia op. cit., p. 771.

30 Liz Carmichael, 14 February 2004; Yehuda Kaplan in a letter to Simonne Horwitz, 4 May 2005; Hunt op. cit., p. 23.

31 D Saffer and G Modi (1994) 'Neurology'. In A Dubb and K Huddle (eds) *Baragwanath Hospital: 50 Years, A Medical Miscellany.* Johannesburg: Department of Medicine, Baragwanath Hospital, p. 117.

32 Segal et al. op. cit., p. 17.

33 Frack (1970) op. cit., pp. 183–240.

34 Hunt op. cit., pp. 1–4.

35 Frack op. cit., p. 208.

36 'Angry Old Man Asks Why? Why? Why?', *Rand Daily Mail*, 5 November 1963; 'Baragwanath Hospital Appointment', *Sunday Express*, 5 April 1964.

37 André Giraud, 12 July 2004. For more on the nurses' response to these events see Chapter 4.

38 'Dead Youth was Shot, Says Doctor', *Rand Daily Mail*, 17 June 1976.

39 Hunt op. cit., p. 254; 'Fear Drives White Doctors from Soweto', *Rand Daily Mail*, 10 January 1977; Moira Russell in a letter to Simonne Horwitz, 6 April 2004; Beukes op. cit., p. 55.

40 D Blumsohn (1994) 'The Pathology of Poverty'. In K Huddle and A Dubb (eds) *Baragwanath Hospital: 50 Years, A Medical Miscellany.* Johannesburg: Department of Medicine, Baragwanath Hospital, pp. 7–13.

41 Helen Rees, 26 July 2004; Effie Shultz, 7 July 2004; Yehuda Kaplan, 1 March 2004.

42 Max Price, 30 August 2004; 'Birdshot Victims Shun Police-guarded Bara', *Weekly Mail*, 25 October 1985. The Truth and Reconciliation Commission of South Africa: Final Report (Cape Town, 1998), Vol. 4, Chapter 5, paragraph 35 gives evidence of the police seizing and using hospital records to identify activists.

43 Digby (2005) op. cit., pp. 452–3.

44 This anti-apartheid movement, formed in the 1950s under the leadership of the ANC, brought together the Congresses of the Indian and coloured peoples, the mostly white Congress of Democrats and the South African Congress of Trade Unions (SACTU).

45 See also Kaplan papers, 'Doctor Who Mixed with Non-Whites is Sacked', *Sunday Times* (no date) and Kaplan to Dr Eleanor Ettlinger, secretary of the Medical Committee against Racial Discrimination in South Africa, London, 23 November 1960.

46 Effie Shultz, 7 July 2004; Truth and Reconciliation Commission of South Africa: Final Report (Cape Town 1998), Vol. 4, Chapter 5, paragraph 34; Baldwin-Ragaven et al. op. cit.

47 Timol was a sportsman and teacher who studied in Moscow in the late 1960s before returning to South Africa to help rebuild the underground structures of the revolutionary movement. He was arrested on 22 October 1971. Five days later he was murdered in the notorious John Vorster Square police station in Johannesburg; his body was badly mutilated. See I Cajee (2005) *Timol – Quest for Justice: Ahmed Timol's Life and Martyrdom*, Johannesburg: STE.

48 Black Consciousness leader Steve Biko died in detention in 1977 at the hands of the South African police. His death and the subsequent investigation raised critical and ethical issues about the conduct of the doctors responsible for his care and about the subsequent response of the medical profession as a whole. See GR McLean and T Jenkins (2003) 'The Steve Biko Affair: A Case Study in Medical Ethics', *Developing World Bioethics*, 3:1 (May), pp. 77–95.

49 Cited in CW Bell (1998) 'World's Largest Hospital Juggles Limited Resources to Deliver Adequate Care'. *Modern Healthcare* 28, p. 1. A similar point was made by Reg Broekman, 27 July 2004.

50 Liz Carmichael, 14 February 2004. See also L Carmichael (2004) *Friendship: Interpreting Christian Love*, London: T & T Clark, which deals with her experiences of multiracial friendship in apartheid South Africa within a spiritual, theological and philosophical framework.

51   Beukes op. cit., p. 9.

52   M Jarrett-Kerr (1961) *African Pulse: Scenes from an African Hospital Window*. London: Morehouse-Barlow, p. 113.

53   Chris van den Heever, 6 October 2004. St John's College is an elite private church school in Johannesburg and King David High School is one of Johannesburg's Jewish day schools.

54   '... and you will remain a 'Bara Boetie.'

55   Beukes op. cit., p. 7.

56   Beukes op. cit., pp. 13–4.

57   'Bara Boetie Cartoon' from Bara PR Archives, *Barameter*, July 1988.

58   The term does not seem to be gender specific and I heard people refer to women as 'Bara Boeties'.

CHAPTER 5

Black Nurses in White
The Nurses of Baragwanath Hospital[1]

To lighten the darkness of ill health over Africa is the wide vision which
Baragwanath Hospital has for its nurses. This is depicted in its badge
which shows a radiant lamp, the symbol of nursing, casting light over
the whole continent. This can be true if all service given in this great
hospital springs from real desire to serve the sick with kindness and
gentleness, as well as with efficiency and good organisation.[2]

These words of Wendy Petersen, senior principal of the Baragwanath
Nursing College from 1954 to 1963, capture the way that the white
nursing establishment and hospital administration characterised the role of
black nurses in South Africa. The notion that nurses would bring to the world
not only good health but also 'light' – which here implies a Western-educated
outlook – runs through the history of black nursing in South Africa and across
the continent. Nursing was one of the most important avenues for African
women to enter paid employment and find independent careers yet very little
has been written on the history of nursing in South Africa; about how black
nurses saw their role; what inspired and motivated them; their perspectives
on nursing; or how nurses functioned within the hospital system during
apartheid.[3] This chapter shows the important role that nurses played in the
history of Baragwanath. Nurses were the backbone of the hospital, the most
numerous of the staff, and a group without whom all services at the hospital
would have ground to a halt. A focused discussion of nurses at Baragwanath
brings the voices of individual, mostly black, nurses to the fore and gives us
insight into how they acted in the contradictory settings of the apartheid state.
Within structures that sought to oppress black people, especially women,
nursing offered them access to the labour market and increasing status
and responsibility, albeit as part of the framework of racial segregation and
separate development. The number of black nurses at Baragwanath continued
to rise throughout the apartheid era.

Table 2: Number of nurses at Baragwanath, 1947–1968[4]

Staff Category[5]		1947	1952	1957	1962	1968
Matrons	White	3	7	22	24	20
	Black	–	–	–	7	12
Sisters	White	33	38	–	–	–
	Black	2	6	35	38	88
Staff-nurses	White	–	–	–	–	–
	Black	118	120	221	304	471
Student-nurses	White	–	–	–	–	–
	Black	240	397	500 (249 in pre-nursing course)	660	668
Student-midwives	White	–	–	–	–	–
	Black	–	–	–	95	200

The growth in numbers continued in the 1970s (by 1982 there were over 4 000 black nurses at the hospital and its primary health care clinics) and until the mid-1980s, when Baragwanath had 23 per cent of its general nursing posts and 16 per cent of its obstetrical nursing posts frozen even as patient numbers continued to rise.

Why black women entered nursing: The Baragwanath experience

In the late 1950s a questionnaire was given to thirty-five Baragwanath students to ascertain their motivations for entering nursing. The results are illustrated in Figure 2:

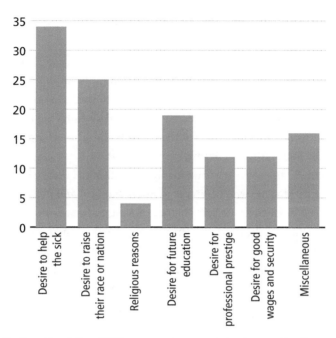

Figure 3: Results of the 1950s survey to ascertain the motivations of women entering nurses' training at Baragwanath Hospital

The motivations of women entering nursing begin to show us the ways in which they formulated their identity as part of a broader sisterhood of nurses and as 'Bara nurses'. The survey offered a useful framework with which to examine how young women expressed their motivations, but without knowing more about the survey it is difficult to know if the nurses were ranking existing categories or expressing their own opinions. Nurses I spoke to identified 'altruistic motivations' and the 'desire for an increase in status' as significant, and these reasons were also prominent in nurses' own writings. At the same time, professional prestige appeared of fundamental importance. Nurses did not talk about 'professional prestige' as such; rather, it showed up in the way nurses spoke about their uniform, homes, and social class. Many nurses also mentioned the importance of factors not highlighted by this survey, such as the limited options black women had for pursuing a professional career and the fact that nurses' training was paid for by the state.

Exploring the 'altruistic' motivations for entering nursing

For many nurses, as for many doctors, the health care profession was one to which they felt called. Some felt it was a religious calling while others felt it was a more general call to heal and to help those in distress. These philanthropic motivations linked Baragwanath's black nurses to the generally accepted, broader universal ideals of the nurses' calling and also played out in a specifically South African context.

The humanitarian aspect of nursing was ably summed up by a semi-retired sister, Matilda Mogale, who had worked in the medical and maternity wards at Baragwanath for three decades before moving to Baragwanath's primary health care clinics: 'I grew up with this thing in me that said I wanted to help other people, especially the sick and the helpless, and maybe make a difference in their lives'. Mpe Tenza, who had grown up in Soweto, and did her training at a mission hospital in the Free State before returning to Baragwanath in the early 1970s, recounted how her mother had told her that as a child she loved to take care of people. 'I was not afraid of taking care of wounds'; she always knew she would be a nurse. For these nurses humanitarian motives were linked to helping people. The race or socio-economic status of the patients did not seem to enter into the discussion as it did for many of the doctors. In the interviews I conducted, doctors often linked humanitarian motives to working at a hospital and serving the black population. For the nurses who, prior to the late 1970s had little choice but to work at a black hospital, altruism did not seem to be linked to any particular site or type of hospital.

Interestingly, the older nurses commented on the changes they perceived, over time, in altruism. There seemed to be a feeling among older nurses that the new generation who came into nursing from the late 1970s were no longer doing so out of humanitarianism. Bemoaning the younger nurses, one nursing sister, Florence Mudzuli, looked back and said that 'in those days, whatever profession you took was from the bottom of your heart, you became a nurse because you realised you had to help the people'. Peggy Mohlamme was more direct:

To me it was a calling, the young generation it is not a calling ... now it is not a calling, they want money. We have to force them, the young nurses who are doing a diploma of nursing, we have to force them to do a two-year contract to keep them in the hospitals otherwise they just leave. They go to private clinics or to the UK. The UK just grabs them like I don't know.

Few nurses questioned in the 1950s survey and few nurses whom I interviewed referred to a religious calling to enter nursing. Most of the nurses who stressed the Christian aspect of nursing trained at missionary hospitals. Sister Matilda Mogale, for example, was led to nursing because she felt she had to 'take care of God's children'. Although she was raised in Johannesburg, Mogale decided, in discussion with her priest, to train at a mission hospital. She took up a training position at Jane Furse, in what was then the Northern Transvaal, in 1956. She then returned to Baragwanath where she worked in the wards for three decades before specialising in HIV/AIDS nursing in the 1990s. For nurses like Mogale, Baragwanath was a markedly unchristian place:

> If you come from a Christian family and you go through this training [at a mission hospital] that reminds you of Christianity all the time and then you have to move from that and adapt to a non-Christian environment, a place without a common outlook ... you had to work through adaptation.

While Christian values were important motivating factors for some nurses, in the Baragwanath context they were personal, and not a prominent part of the public narrative as they might be at a mission hospital.

The other humanitarian motivation mentioned in the 1950s survey was, in the words of the survey, 'the desire to raise their race or nation'. For decades, the missionaries, colonialists and nursing administrations stressed that nurses were the 'harbingers of progress'.[6] Many also saw nurses, with the scientific grounding their training in biomedicine brought, as an important link in the eradication of 'backward' traditional beliefs. It was thought that nurses, who were separated from their communities and (in the minds of the authorities) uplifted by their training and their contact with science and technology, could play an important role in the eradication of 'witchcraft' and suspicion. It was hoped that they would act as a conduit for the introduction of western values to African communities. Some in the nursing establishment, such as Charlotte Searle, also espoused this view. In her writing, nursing was an important part of the 'civilising mission', which would 'uplift' black South Africans in a number of ways, including the 'conquering' of 'witchcraft' through scientific medicine.[7] From the quote that begins this chapter it is evident that Petersen saw nursing in a similar light, suggesting that nurses would bring 'light' and education not only to the hospital and the surrounding community but also to the whole continent.[8]

Similar views were expressed by Grace Mashaba, who suggested that 'the black nurse became an influential and prestigious woman in her society, much sought after as a marriage partner. She was, therefore, in a position to set the pace and steer the course of her people's development.'[9] Mashaba often referred in her writings to the idea of nurses uplifting their people:

> The nurses' training for black students was significant in that it was educationally enlightening, socially uplifting and economically advancing for black people in general, and for black women in particular. The foundation was thus laid not only for black nurses to be given academic opportunities but also for a massive campaign against culturally induced ill health.[10]

Mashaba saw nursing as part of a 'civilising project' that would uplift not only the nurse (by teaching her modern western ways) but, through her, her community which would be educated. The very title of Mashaba's book, *Rising to the Challenge of Change*, is imbued with the idea of nurses 'rising' up to face the challenges and to better themselves. While Mashaba's book mirrors earlier triumphalist accounts of nursing in South Africa and elsewhere, it does so from a different position of cultural awareness. As a black nurse, Mashaba gave a unique and valuable history of black nursing in South Africa. Published at a time of hope and liberation, as South Africa stood on the brink of a new country, the book offers a validation of black nurses' roles in the leadership of the profession.

In contrast to the writing of Mashaba, and the accounts of white nurses, interviews with the Baragwanath nurses suggest a more muted attitude towards success by black nurses. This was, perhaps, in part the response of nurses who had been in the hospital for many decades and who had experienced the overcrowded, harsh realities of the wards. For many, even those who rose to positions at the apex of nursing, their individual journeys were marked by hardship, segregation, and challenges.

Even while black nurses were fighting for recognition within the nursing structures, they were seen to play an important role in uplifting their families.

Many women saw nursing as a sophisticated, professional job that would increase their status in the community. A 1970s study of social mobility in an urban community on the Witwatersrand shows how wives in general, but particularly nurses, could influence their husbands' social status. 'A wife could be a very important status symbol and co-earner. The wife of an upper-class Reeftowner therefore, must ideally be not only educated but professional, not a teacher but a nurse and preferably a staff nurse'.[11]

The same seems to have held true at Baragwanath, at least in the public narrative. An article celebrating Baragwanath's twenty-first birthday cites the hospital's matron suggesting that nurses were sought-after marriage partners because nursing 'fits a young girl with the qualities that she will need when she is a woman, qualities needed in a wife and mother'.[12] Whatever the reason, many nurses married professionals who were teachers, academics, religious leaders, traditional leaders, lawyers, or medical practitioners. Peggy Francina Mohlamme, the first black matron of the maternity section at Baragwanath, was married to Professor Jacob Mohlamme, the first black South African to gain a PhD in African History, which he received from the University of Wisconsin in 1985. Dora Nginza was married to an Eastern Cape chief. Other nurses were married to, and were themselves, prominent leaders in the anti-apartheid struggle. Albertina Sisulu trained as a nurse at the Non-European Hospital before the opening of Baragwanath. Her future husband, prominent ANC and anti-apartheid activist Walter Sisulu, was the brother of a fellow nurse. Adelaide Tambo, wife of Oliver Tambo, worked as a nurse at Baragwanath in the late 1950s. Maggie Resha trained as a nurse at a mission hospital in Pondoland (in the late 1950s Resha was one of the driving forces behind the nurses' strike at Baragwanath Hospital).[13] Nelson Mandela's first wife Edith Ntoko was also a nurse. Although not a nurse, his second wife Winnie Madikizela-Mandela, began working at Baragwanath as a social worker after graduating in 1956. The social standing of being a nurse, or being married to one, seems to have bolstered their social and political credibility. Baragwanath became something of a space for elite social and political networking among and for African women, as much as it was for doctors.

Exploring status-linked motives for entering nursing

The 1950s survey offered three reasons linked to an uplifting of status for young women wanting to enter nursing. The first was 'a desire for further education'; the second 'a desire for good wages and security'; and the third an all-embracing category of 'professional prestige', although these categories were often difficult to separate in nurses' own ways of talking about their motives.

Twelve of the 1950s survey respondents mentioned good wages and security as reasons for going into nursing. Further investigation into nursing, wages and money reveals a more complex picture. Firstly, black women had few professional career options in apartheid South Africa: they were largely restricted to teaching or nursing. Therefore, discussions about black women in the professions have to take into account limited opportunities. The nurses interviewed were acutely aware of these limitations. Florence Mudzuli: 'I got my matric in 1952, I thought I must go to high school and from there into nursing. Again, in those years there were not many other professions available to us and I come from the Free State, where we did not know about many other professions, the education was not so good.'

Nursing had a distinct financial advantage over teaching during the training phase. Student nurses did not pay fees or for accommodation at their training hospital and they got paid during their training. For many, this was a deciding factor. Harriet Gwebu, who trained at Baragwanath during the late 1960s: 'Nursing was actually my second choice. My first choice was teaching, but my parents could not send me to university so I went for my second choice ... where we got paid [while training].' Years later, Gwebu managed to combine nursing and teaching when, after working in the Obstetrics, Surgery and the Intensive Care Units at Baragwanath, she became a tutor at the Baragwanath Nursing College in the early 1990s. For Albertina Sisulu, money was also a deciding factor: 'I wanted to be a teacher. But conditions wouldn't allow me to be a teacher. So I had to take up nursing, where when you are training you are being paid. So my hope was that at least if I am being paid, I will be able to help my brothers and sister.'[14] In her book *Their Light, Love and Life: A Black Nurse's Story* Ntsoaki Senokoanyane tells the semi-autobiographical story of Busi, a young girl entering nurses' training just as she did herself.

I never intended to be a nurse. Unlike many young black girls, who dream of the smart uniform and the status offered by nursing, I saw it as a job where one spent one's time doing unpleasant tasks for sick people. My ambition was to be a social worker. But higher education was out of the question for our family. My father, who had only studied up to Standard Five, was very anxious that his children should be educated, but how do you educate ten children on a workman's wage? Bursaries appeared to be only for children of people like teachers, principals and school inspectors. If you were a poor man's child, nursing was – and still is – the only answer, because this way you earn while you are training and do not have to pay fees.[15]

The advantage of being paid wages during training should not be taken to indicate that black nurses were satisfied with their financial rewards. Once they were qualified, the nurses' salaries were low, and some nurses complained about the salaries in interviews, pointing out that they did not enter the profession for the money. Florence Mudzuli, who started training in 1956:

Point number one our salaries were very low. You will not believe it. In 1966 we were £1.99 per month, that was for first six months and then we were registered and we got £13. What is that? R26 per month. As a double qualified nurse you could get £39 per month. But because those days, whatever profession you took was from the bottom of your heart, you became a nurse because you realised you had to help the people, so salary was not a problem to us ... it was beautiful. You enjoy it.

Mudzuli's recollection of the salary seems impossibly low (but the salient point is that a high salary was not always what attracted women to the profession). Data for black nurses' salaries from 1966 to 1978[16] shows that while senior matrons' and ward sisters' salaries rose during the decade they were quickly eroded by inflation so that they were very similar at the end of the 1970s to what they had been a decade earlier. Sisters' salaries in 1969 were between R840 and R1 200, rising to between R1 740 and R1 980 by 1974 (R1 177 to R1 340 in 1969 currency), and R1 740 to R2 100 (R989 to R1 153 in 1969 currency) in 1976.[17] Among staff nurses, the raises in the early 1970s were not as large, so their salaries were more rapidly eroded by inflation, even by the mid-1970s. Throughout the period however, nurses' salaries reflected their professional status. Black mineworkers' salaries were R199 in 1969 and rose to R636 in 1974.[18] This was, however, only around one-third of that of a sister and also significantly less than staff nurses' salaries, which by then started at over R900 – even when the nursing profession was predominantly made up of female workers.

Black nurses were aware that their salaries differed vastly from the salaries of their white counterparts. Florence Mudzuli:

> There had always been unfairness in the sense that even salaries and treatments were not the same. Everything was not the same! So you can imagine, you train with a white nurse and you complete at the same time but once you become a registered nurse then the discrepancy is so much. You remain black with your black salary and she remains white with her white salary.

Although there were always differences in the salaries of white, coloured, Indian and black nurses, the gap widened dramatically in the 1960s. By the end of the decade black nurses were earning about forty-five per cent of their white counterparts' salary.[19] Nonetheless, the salary differential did not seem to dissuade women from entering the profession. Disempowered as they were by the white-dominated hierarchy and the professional bodies, there was little they could do about it. Decision-making, for African women, seemed to be based more on the fact that, of the limited opportunities available to them, nursing offered an independent income and financial assistance during training. Job security was also fairly certain at this time, with a constant need for nurses.[20] However, these points alone cannot explain their reasons for entering nursing. Another of the motives mentioned in the survey was 'the desire for further education'.

Post-secondary education for black women in apartheid South Africa was limited. The fairly stringent entrance qualifications associated with nursing meant that simply being accepted into training was a mark of educational achievement. To enter nurses' training in the late 1940s and 1950s a young woman had to obtain a minimum of a Junior Certificate (ten years of schooling). In 1963 the South African Nursing Council (SANC) decided that a Matric Certificate (thirteen years of schooling for black learners) was the baseline for admission.[21] From the end of the 1970s, the Matric Certificate, now twelve years of schooling, was still the basis of acceptance.

Many nurses were proud of their education and, when asked to recount their nursing careers during interviews, stressed periods when they had taken additional degrees and diplomas. At reunions and graduations of Baragwanath nurses, those from various generations wore their academic gowns and degree hoods. Those with multiple degrees proudly wore multiple hoods.

Nurses were also attracted to nursing by the education they gained through training and the independence that this education gave them in the medical arena. For one sister, Florence Mudzuli, who was raised in the Free State and did her initial training at the first hospital that accepted her, Coronation, going into nursing was a decision motivated by this perceived independence:

> It was my father's influence ... My father used to work in the mines and trained as a first aid person and when I grew up I found him running a mine hospital by himself. The doctor only came once a week and he would only be referring cases that he could not manage or cases that he thought were serious ... I always thought my father was a doctor because he was doing everything independently in the mines and from there I like nursing.

Many of the Baragwanath nurses who served as nurse-practitioners in the primary health clinics expressed similar thoughts. For them it was not the extra degree they earned by doing the post-basic course but the fact that, as Matilda Mogale said, 'out there you get to use your brain.' Mpe Tenza, who had been working in the wards at Baragwanath for a decade when she was seconded to the clinics, explained how her attitude towards her new role changed:

> When they told me I had to go I did not like it. I thought, that is doctors' stuff, it did not excite me. I want to nurse a patient ... I completed PHC (Primary Health Care) and I found there is still patient contact but you make your own decisions ... In the wards it was doctor first and then you carried out the orders. In the clinics you took the initiative of what to do now because the doctor is not on duty so it is really exciting.

Some of Tenza's reluctance to move to the clinics could have been rooted in ideas about the educational value of clinic work. For example, when Virginia Ramogale, who trained at Baragwanath in the early 1980s, wanted to move to the clinics shortly after qualifying, she encountered antagonism from some of her peers at the hospital:

> The feeling was that very few young nurses wanted to go to the clinics. They would say that there are elderly people there and you should get experience here. They thought that the hospital was providing more knowledge and that at the clinics were old, outdated people. That was different from what I experienced because I gained more knowledge, more than the profession itself there.

In the clinics nurses were able to interact more directly with patients, often with no doctor present. Many nurses thought that these encounters benefited from mutual cultural understandings of illness. This was particularly so for Margaret Mohlala, who had begun her training at Baragwanath in 1955. She continued to work there, furthering her education with a course in paediatric nursing in 1973, and in 1977 she trained as a nurse-clinician.

> When you do a consultation you pick up that people are happy to see you because you are from the community ... they see you not so much as a nurse but as one of them. They know that you understand what you are talking about ... For instance, a patient would come in and say, 'You know sister I think that I am suffering from *inyongo*'. When you say you are suffering from *inyongo* we know because we were also told at our own homes that when you have eaten a lot of sweets you have *inyongo*. You are given some castor oil or whatever is available to clean the bowel. And they will tell you that they have given themselves an enema ... They might say I need an African herb, but you see, because we are now trained and we understand better, as a health worker you go back to this enema and the African herb things and you educate the patient. You make it known that you are not condemning the African herbs on principle. There are differences between the African herbs and the western type of enema. You also say you can get complications like renal shutdown sometimes, not because the herb is wrong but because the herb it is just not right to use then. These are what the things are that make the person feel free to interact with them because they know you understand what they are talking about.

In these encounters nurses were able to bridge two medical worlds; to use their knowledge of both systems of healing to attend to and educate patients. They saw the kind of medicine practised in the clinics as of great value to the patient and rewarding for themselves, and that this type of work offered a different educational experience that allowed them to develop their sense of independence.

The final category in the 1950s survey of nurses' motivations was 'a desire for professional prestige'. While only twelve of the respondents in the survey mentioned this as a motivation for entering nursing, for many of the nurses in my study professional prestige, in one form or another, was important. It was also the professional image of nursing that, more than anything else, linked the Baragwanath nurses to nursing's broader sisterhood. For many nurses, black and white, professional prestige was intrinsically linked to the view of nursing as a profession of dignified, sophisticated and caring women. Nursing was also seen as a profession in which women worked with advanced technology, something which brought them added respect. Many of the ideas around professional prestige showed up in the nurses' own ways of talking about dress, deportment, and status. For example, Mpe Tenza:

> There was another motivation for me becoming a nurse. At a later age when I was in high school, we used to visit our friends' sisters there and when we entered the gates of Baragwanath the picture we saw of the nurses there, it was just a poster you know. [SH: can you explain what you mean?] It was beautiful; they were so clean, sterile. Everything was just perfect, the way they walked in those corridors of Baragwanath, and we just told our peers that this is the right profession for us. Then when we went to see the sick patients in the wards as visitors and we would see them walking in those wards, very, very straight, bright and shaking the thermometers like this [she demonstrates] ... that was another motivation for us. We used to visit the nurses' home during their off duty time, so when we got there we found them busy, some were reading magazines, some books, other were doing hand work, crocheting and I said this is the profession for me.

Peggy Francina Mohlamme told how she had grown up with her grandmother who encouraged her to be a nurse, saying that her hands made old people feel comfortable. Later, when she was living with her aunt near Coronation

Hospital in Newclare, Johannesburg, she had the opportunity to observe the nurses at the hospital:

> Me and two of my friends would walk to Cora just to watch the nurses, and those days the nurses were putting on red and white,[22] and that used to make me feel so good about nurses. They were so tidy, their caps were nice and clean and the wearing of stockings was another story – fascinating! And the shoes were shining you know and that made me feel very good about the nurses. Actually we used to go in casualty to watch, like naughty little boys without permission, and we would see this girl coming in at two o'clock and doing these things only to discover it was a thermometer. We would see her doing it all the time with the thermometer and it was fascinating and we felt so good about that. We were three friends and two of us decided, how about becoming nurses ... Eventually we had to qualify for nursing.

Mohlamme qualified at a mission hospital and came to Baragwanath as a staff nurse in the early 1960s. She went on to do her post-basic training at Baragwanath and climbed through the ranks, eventually being appointed to the post of matron of the Baragwanath Maternity Hospital in the mid-1980s and in 1993 became chief nursing service manager (formally chief matron). For Mohlamme, nursing gave young women a sense of self pride and dignity. As a young women she was also impressed by the ways in which nurses used biomedical such as the thermometers.

In nurses' portrayal of their own identities one of the overwhelming themes was that of cleanliness, dress and style – especially in connection with the nurses' uniform. Many nurses saw the uniform as a symbol of personal status and professional prestige. One nurse, who completed her training at Baragwanath in 1976, explained that she held ambitions of being a nurse in part because she 'was attracted by them walking along the street, in the white spotless uniform'. Another nurse, who grew up in Sekhukuneland, spoke about how, as a child, she admired the white uniforms of the nurses she saw at Jane Furse. Mia Brandel-Syrier's 1953 investigation among the nurses of a large black hospital on the Reef found that several answers to the question 'how did you get the idea of becoming a nurse?' revolved around similar issues. Many suggested that 'they had *seen* other nurses who 'were smart', 'looked important', 'apparently earned a lot of money', or who had, in other ways, impressed them and had made them desire to become like them.[23] In her autobiography, Resha also recalls being impressed by the smartly dressed nurses she saw around her and being charmed by their kindness and cleanliness.[24] The focus on cleanliness is significant because this was in sharp contrast to the white perception of the African body as diseased and dirty; nurses strove, perhaps subconsciously, to be the exact opposite of this offensive stereotype. They were sophisticated, well-educated women who were not only well dressed but wore starched white uniforms – the ultimate public display of hygiene and cleanliness. They were careful to portray themselves as modern individuals at the cutting edge of modernity through their knowledge of hospital equipment and their thoroughly professional dress. The uniform was more than merely a symbol of belonging to a profession. It was also a symbol of class and status, as Mpe Tenza, one nurse, remembered nostalgically: 'The uniform was so smart, that is what created dignity with the nurses.' Florence Mudzuli: 'It was the respect. You know nurses were respected in the community. When you pass, when you walk in your white uniform even the children knew that there is a nurse passing.' In a world where black South Africans, especially women, were facing increasing discrimination, the dignity symbolised by the uniform and the respect nurses gained in the community were important factors in drawing women to nursing.

Many nurses had role models who were nurses. For Mohlala it was 'a district midwife, visiting homes and washing babies'. Similarly, for Elsina Totsa: 'There was a nurse where I was, who had trained at Baragwanath, she was in charge of the clinic next to the school. She was nice looking, having those white dresses and a veil and she used to care for her patients. She was a kind lady and she made me wish to do the job she was doing.' Totsa's role model led her not only into nursing but also to Baragwanath.

The way that nurses dressed and presented themselves was not altogether removed from ideas of patient care. Mpe Tenza, a highly qualified nurse with a Master's degree in nursing administration, thought that 'as a nurse when you come to a sick patient's bed, she or he lifts up his eyes and expects to see some glowing person'. The clean and beautiful nurse, she went on to explain, is an important part of patient care. In her book dealing with the life story of an African nurse, Senokoanyane gives an example of a patient's reaction to the nurse in her uniform: 'I saw this little nurse in a beautiful white dress, and from the manner in which she greeted me I could sense that here is Jesus ... and she did help me'.[25] In a letter of thanks to Matron McLarty, the husband of a Baragwanath patient wrote that his wife 'paints such a vivid picture of your love and tenderness to her as reminds one of a Florence Nightingale'.[26] Here, the nurse's image linked by the patient to the classic image of the lady nurse, and through this image to the broader sisterhood of nurses. A final example, a poem, 'The Queen-like Sister of Ward Twelve' written by Joe Tshabalala, a sixty-four-year old patient in Baragwanath's paraplegic ward, also suggests that the patients respected the nurses and saw their style and demeanour as important:

Yes, if it were that all sisters
Were good, human and really
Kind, I would have them all
Properly told that to follow the
Example of the ward twelve
Sister was the goal the world
Seeks for, without seeking for
This goal none will be as good
As this human example. Her gait
Is slow-sharp and ladily and
Interestingly very natural. Her figure
Leanish, effable indeed she is,
Respectful and respectable in her
Personality and very considerate
With regards to her patients.
Pretty features she has and that's
What commands her self respect.[27]

It was not only dress that created the idealised image of the nurse. Even in their spare time nurses looked for activities symbolising modernity, prestige and social influence.[28] The activities the Baragwanath nurses undertook during their free time were those activities of an educated urban elite: reading and doing handwork. Margaret Mohlala, who lived near Edenvale Hospital when she was young, talked about seeing nurses doing ballroom dancing near her house: 'One day we decided to go to the hall and see what was taking place there. We found these nurses, so beautiful and taking dance lessons. More and more and more I developed that love for nursing. When I left school already I knew I wanted to do nursing, so that is how I started.'

The emphasis on style, image and class seemed to permeate all aspects of a nurse's training. When asked about what she remembered most about her training at Baragwanath during the early 1980s, Virginia Ramogale spoke about how young trainee nurses were taught to appear professional so that they could act professionally:

> I can remember our tutor when we came in there. She was a real motivation for us. She said 'at month-end you are going to be paid and you should buy yourselves some school bags. I don't want any plastic. You must not use toilet paper to wipe your nose or you will not be a lady. You must buy yourselves a pair of stockings and then you must be a real lady.' And immediately on month-end I was up and about to buy those things. You know when you start, they say take out your book and you are scratching for them it is not professionalism ... Having these things, it made us look like we were ladies and you should look in a professional way.

It was not only the nurses who were expected to dress respectably. Anna Montso said of one of her tutors, 'She wanted us to be neat all the time, and even our boyfriends! We must not have boyfriends who do not look presentable'.

Commenting on the general atmosphere in the nursing college, Ramogale pointed out: 'Now you felt that at least you were someone and that pride that you are doing something and you are being recognised as an adult, it was such a good feeling'. Elsina Totsa: 'The nurses' home, it was wonderful. We had a caretaker from the hospital to look after the rooms and make things clean. Our laundry was done by the hospital and food-wise it was good'. The nurses home provided modern amenities and inspired dignity. It was a place where they felt at home. 'She [a tutor] would say treat this place like your home, it was nice', recalled Annah Montso.

These idealised images were not the only interpretation of life as a student nurse. For some nurses the training facilities were a very nurturing environment but for others the atmosphere was very paternalistic. Nurses had to get permission to visit their homes and were told when they had to be back. Visitors, especially male visitors, were monitored. Margaret Mohlala, who remembers being escorted by her father to Johannesburg to start her nursing training at Baragwanath at the age of seventeen, also remembered her father being impressed by the rules at the nurses' quarters:

> We could have visitors to 6 pm then after that no visitors. This security guy who used to stand at Bara's front view at the time ... would actually even get visitors out of the sitting room on his way to the gate even before six. If he walked past at quarter to six he would just come in ... and he would say 'Bakwenyana', which means 'sons-in-law', it is time for you to go, it was just like that!

Anastasia Zungu spoke about the harsh experiences she endured: 'The sisters were too militaristic! As a junior you had to dance to the music of that power, not for the patients. Once at Bara I was doing a bed-pan when the matron called me to do something else but I finished with the patient, and the sister said to me "who is more important me or the patient?" and I said "the patient". Eish! I got a bad report!'

While nurses might have had differing reasons for taking up the profession, the status that nursing gave them and the ways in which they present themselves united them. They prioritised a set of shared professional ideals linking South African nurses to what McLarty called 'the great sisterhood of nurses both nationally and internationally'.[29] Yet, black South African nurses never wholly belonged to this 'universal' sisterhood. Excluded from positions of leadership in nursing associations and isolated in a black hospital, nurses at Baragwanath negotiated an identity drawing on universal stereotypical images but also rooted in the local Baragwanath experience.

The Baragwanath experience and identity

In the quote that began this chapter Petersen referred to Baragwanath as 'this great hospital'. The idea of Baragwanath as a special and even unique place was often repeated by the hospital administration, by doctors and by nurses and the image was to some extent shaped and reinforced by the hospital administration. The government often painted Baragwanath as their showpiece, printing stories and photographs of nurses – always immaculately dressed and smiling – in government-sponsored publications. These articles stressed the contribution that the state and provincial administration made to the training of black nurses to equip them to serve their own people, thereby serving the goals of separate development.[30] The popular media also presented this image. For example, an article on the occasion of Baragwanath's twenty-first birthday commented that 'perhaps more than anything else Baragwanath, as no other hospital in South Africa, has placed non-white nursing on a sound footing'.[31]

The nursing sector portrayed a similar image of Baragwanath and its nurses. One of the few black nurses to write about the history of nursing in South Africa, Grace Mashaba, wrote that Baragwanath 'was to become the show-piece of black nurses' training and development in the Transvaal'. She went on to comment that 'Baragwanath school was clearly a shining example of the best and most enterprising of schools for black nurses'. McLarty spoke proudly of how Baragwanath was known internationally for nursing achievement. Baragwanath's white nursing administration, matrons and tutors also stressed the special nature of nursing training at Baragwanath as their articles on the tenth and twenty-first anniversaries of the founding of the hospital demonstrate.[32] These articles stress the quality of Baragwanath's nurses, the unique aspects of their training, and their dedication to their patients.

The black nurses at Baragwanath often spoke about the hospital in similar terms. Looking back on her career at Baragwanath Matilda Mogale commented: 'It was very special, it was special in the service, especially in the doctors and nurses.' During interviews and in informal conversations, nurses often stressed a similar sentiment to that of Margaret Mohlala who pointed out that 'Bara at the time was a very famous hospital'. It was, in the words of Virginia Ramogale, 'one of *the* hospitals. When you trained at Bara you knew that at least it was a recognised hospital, known everywhere. The standards of teaching were very high so everybody from the surrounding area wanted specifically to come to Bara'. Others came to Baragwanath because they were influenced by role models. For still others, there was a family connection to the hospital. Mpe Tenza: 'I knew Baragwanath from a very young age, and my older sister was a nursing assistant, one of the very first nurses who was appointed at Bara.' Still others came because of the perceived distinctiveness of its training. Mashaba suggests that the 'positive, humanistic and broad-minded outlook must have contributed to the high standard of nurses' training at Baragwanath Hospital'.[33] Important figures in the early training of nurses at Baragwanath, such as McLarty and Petersen, played a significant role in setting the educational philosophy at the hospital, strongly discouraging rote-learning, which was common in many training hospitals at the time, especially among nurses whose first language was not English. Students at Baragwanath were encouraged to do independent studies, use the library provided for them, and record case histories.[34]

Baragwanath integrated a number of specific courses into the training programme, including orientation programmes for new staff that aimed to help the nurse 'find her place in this enormous institution'.[35] This went some way towards welcoming new nurses and introducing them to the Baragwanath ways. There was also a study course of several months' duration, 'The role and responsibility of the trained staff in this institution'. The course enabled staff to gain insight into their own work and that of their colleagues. It was designed to stimulate nurses' interest in further study and promotion. Such courses, together with the pre-nursing course discussed earlier, could also have focused nurses' attention on the opportunities Baragwanath provided and brought their identities as Baragwanath nurses to the fore.

The image of Baragwanath nurses, as well as their perceptions of the distinctive training the hospital provided, seems to have played a role in some nurses' choice of training school and their construction of a Baragwanath identity. However, not all nurses who ended up at Baragwanath had chosen to train there and some who spent most of their careers at Baragwanath had trained elsewhere. Before exploring this aspect in more detail, it is worth pointing out that in the context of black nursing in South Africa, the word 'choice' needs to be qualified as there were limited options available for black nurses. In Johannesburg, for example, Coronation Hospital was an option but by the 1960s it was focused on training and recruiting coloured nurses. One Baragwanath nurse, Florence Mudzuli, who had trained at Coronation between 1956 and 1960, explained:

> I remember when they were recruiting coloured nurses for Cora, the white matron that we had then were coming to people like us – you can see I used to be light in complexion – and she would try to give us an opportunity to become coloured. She would say, from your complexion you look like a coloured, and we can change your surname so you have a coloured surname so we can take you here in our hospital. But you know in those days there was such a lot of racial segregation that you just said, how can I become a coloured when everyone at home is

black? ... Some of us did fall for that, some of them became coloured. We refused and I am so proud, we remained blacks!

Mission hospitals were another training alternative to large provincial hospitals. Some women had religious reasons for choosing mission hospitals; however, others had different reasons. Mpe Tenza said: 'My father wanted me to come to Baragwanath for training and I said no ways! All my sisters and my brothers have been to boarding schools and I am left at home. Every time I am the one who scrubs the floors and does what-what, and so I said no I am getting out, I'm going to a mission!' The mission training schools were, however, often small and some found their applications rejected on the basis that the schools were full. These small, often remote, hospitals also did not offer the same range of training and experience as the larger urban hospitals.[36]

There were nurses who trained at Baragwanath for instrumental reasons. For Virginia Ramogale it was 'the nearest hospital to home'. For others it was close to families, boyfriends or husbands who were living and working in Johannesburg. There were other women, like Margaret Mohlala, who knew very little about the hospital: 'At the time it was just a hospital to me. No-one told me anything about Johannesburg to start with or about Bara. It was just as a student I wanted to find a place where I could train ... I applied all over the country and I got a position at Bara'.

Once at Baragwanath, they found new challenges. The nurses were not a homogeneous group. In the first decade of training at Baragwanath students were predominantly black, with a few coloured and Indian students. They were drawn from all areas of South Africa, with about a quarter of the students from rural areas, a quarter from small towns and the remainder from urban areas.[37] They spoke several different languages. This multilinguistic environment was something that many nurses mentioned in interviews. For Annah Montso, who grew up in the Free State, 'the main interesting thing was the language. You get up in the morning and you find someone speaking Xhosa and Zulu, someone speaking Pretoria-style Tswana, and it was quite thrilling.' When Elsina Totsa took up a position as a staff nurse at Baragwanath in the early 1960s she found she had to learn a new language:

The first few months was hectic, the language spoken was different. The hospital was mostly Sotho speaking and I was Xhosa. I did not understand and I learned it like a course, you just adjusted yourself to be inquisitive and that is how I learned what this and this means and I became fluent in Sotho.

Not everyone agreed that the hospital was mainly Sotho speaking. Anastasia Zungu, who grew up in Sekhukhuneland before coming to Baragwanath in 1959, thought that 'the language was difficult, most people spoke Zulu and we spoke to the community in English'. Language was further complicated by the fact that most of the doctors were white and spoke either English or Afrikaans – and could not, for the most part, speak any African languages. Nurses were often called on to translate. Speaking about her experience in the wards prior to the 1980s Florence Mudzuli said that 'nurses were doing a lot of interpretation ... [the patients] knew that we are their children and we are between them and the doctors. We are going to tell the doctors about them as much as we are going to tell them about the doctors, so we used to be a very good middleman. It was a good position because you had to understand the patient for you to be able to tell the doctor this is what she did because she had to.'

It was also notable that the nurses translated selectively. Harriet Gwebu:

Actually, we would not even tell the doctor if the patient tells you he had consulted a traditional healer because you knew that the patient would get a telling off ... The doctor would be quite unimpressed and say 'why did you go? You see now you have witchdoctor poison' and so the patient would tell you and you say, the doctor will not understand what you are saying, look we better not even mention it.

Nurses valued their position as intermediaries and were able to play a valuable role in mediating the relationship between patients and doctors. The hospital administration also seemed to have been aware of the role they played. For example, one information brochure published during the 1970s suggests that the African nurse 'is keenly aware of the needs of the patient, and she understands the often unspoken but implied fears and anxieties of the Bantu patient. The patient's culture is her culture, and she builds a bridge of understanding between patient and doctor'.[38] It was a similar motivation that led Koos Beukes to call for the training of African nurses to staff the public health clinics. He believed that their knowledge of the language and culture of the people among whom they worked would facilitate health education and better care.[39]

Black nurses who fulfilled the role of translator or intermediary are not unique to Baragwanath. Black nurses at missionary hospitals during the twentieth century worked at the intersection of Western and indigenous medicine, using their knowledge of the systems of Western medicine to educate their communities – and they also acted as brokers of social change.[40] The nurses at Baragwanath recognised that they were drawn from the same community as the patients while the doctors were for the most part outsiders, and in addition many of them felt that Baragwanath's training was superior. Elsina Totsa thought that: 'The training at Bara was quite enlightened. It paved the way. You had more knowledge, more skills. If you trained at Bara they knew you had more skills than other nurses. The basic training, the resources and everything was thorough'. The pride Baragwanath nurses felt in their training and experience was also evident when they recounted stories of coming into contact with nurses from other hospitals. Harriet Gwebu recalled: 'Every time you went to do a course somewhere they would say oh by the way you work at Bara? ... The sentence would always start "Would you tell us what you at Bara do?" because it was felt that we thought we knew more than everybody else, we thought that we were better trained, superior – which we were! And that made us proud.'

Florence Mudzuli remembered that 'the nurses that trained at Bara, whenever they went somewhere for other qualifications they would say "we at Bara do ..." and even outside people knew that if she trained at Bara she was a know-all-nurse. You know, we used to be very smart at Bara.'

The way that the training was structured at Baragwanath was an important factor in their sense of confidence. Nurses often stressed during interviews and in discussions that the practice of having three months of theoretical training before going into the wards gave them a solid grounding and a good balance between practical patient care and theory. This foundation, as well as the post-basic courses offered at the hospital, played an important role in their perception that their training was superior. Baragwanath Hospital, under the leadership of McLarty's successor, Nancy Simpson, was significant in the creation and running of post-basic specialist courses for black nurses.[41] The first course, established in 1959, was in operating theatre technique, and subsequently courses for tutors, orthopaedic nursing, ward administration and intensive care nursing were added.

Whether the training was actually superior at Baragwanath is impossible to ascertain without a comprehensive comparative study of other nurse training institutions. Training was, to some extent, standardised by the South African Nursing Council, which controlled syllabuses. But many of the Baragwanath nurses I interviewed certainly expressed a belief that their training was best, and this was clearly important in creating a confident and positive self-image.

The experience nurses gained in the wards was also an important part of what they interpreted as the Baragwanath experience and ethos. Nurses, like the doctors discussed in the previous chapter, suggested that Baragwanath provided specific opportunities because, as Annah Montso said, 'We have machinery, we have the professors to lecture to the students, the tutors and the nursing sisters in the wards and we do a lot of procedures'. This comment highlights two important things. It points out the benefits that some nurses saw in Baragwanath being a provincial teaching hospital that was well equipped and benefited from the presence of university-linked staff. At the same time it points to the high caseload which provided doctors and nurses with so much experience.

The experience and knowledge the hospital provided was based in part on the epidemiology and in part on the caseloads that presented at the hospital. Florence Mudzuli, echoing the sentiment of many of Baragwanath's doctors, pointed out: 'Just for example, if you are a midwife and you have delivered ten patients, another nurse from outside Bara would have delivered three patients. Those ten would have given you two or three problems that would have made you a good midwife and the problems that you see at Bara as a midwife you might not see at smaller hospitals for a long time.'

As with the doctors, the large patient numbers led nurses to gain a great deal of experience. The volume of cases and the rate of patient turnover must also have increased the pressure on nurses, although that was not a major theme in my interviews with them. During her time as matron, McLarty did note the effects that overcrowding and high patient turnover had on the practice of nursing:

The turnover of patients is much more rapid, convalescent patients have practically vanished from the wards, and there is inevitably less emphasis on the art of nursing. In these conditions it is not surprising that student nurses tend to look on the patient more as a body which is the recipient of frequent injections than a suffering human being in need of the ministration of the nurse. The quickened tempo of the ward also leaves little time either for the trained staff usually insufficient in number, or for the student to practise those small refinements of nursing which means so much to the patient.[42]

Here, McLarty referred to the 1950s. During the decades that followed, as patient numbers increased exponentially, the situation worsened. One nurse pointed out that, especially during the 1970s, the 'shortage of staff was terrible, the pressure was increasing and then increasing'. Referring to the late 1970s, Anastasia Zungu gave the clearest expression of the pressure overcrowding put on the nursing staff. 'The wards were terrible; I did not know what to do. In the paeds ward there were so many children.' However, most nurses stressed the increase of violent trauma rather than the overcrowding.

The perceived distinctiveness of their training and experiences at Baragwanath created a pride in the hospital's nurses and became part of their group identity – not just as nurses but as Baragwanath nurses. Harriet Gwebu thought that Baragwanath 'was the pride of nurses' and spoke about her pride in being a Baragwanath nurse for almost four decades by borrowing the term the doctors use to show their identification with the hospital. She said, 'I was what used to be called a 'Bara Boetie' – a nursing 'Bara Boetie' – and I was proud to be that and I held my head up high.'

Nurses at Baragwanath, like the doctors, perceived there to be a Baragwanath 'group', membership of which was neither easy nor automatic. Mpe Tenza, who did her basic training at a mission hospital in the Free State and then came to Baragwanath to do midwifery, explained how senior nurses advised her of the difficulties she would encounter if she decided to stay and work at Baragwanath:

When I completed one of the senior sisters at Bara said to me, 'you are such a good nurse, but here at Baragwanath, as a person who was not trained here, we are not going to recognise you and give you a senior post. So you should go back'. She was formally trained from where I came from, and she said 'go back to your basic training hospital where you can get promotion'.

Tenza decided to stay at Baragwanath and, having done post-basic courses there and having proved herself in the wards, she was eventually accepted and promoted – by the early 1980s she was serving as a senior tutor at the nursing college. Another nurse who trained at a mission hospital and who encountered suspicion on coming to Baragwanath in 1963 was Peggy Mohlamme:

> When you came from outside Bara they always considered you not to be very up to standard. Especially if you trained at a mission hospital ... You have to work yourself up. You have to demonstrate to them, to say, 'this is who I am and this is what I can do and what I can handle' ... It took me six months and then they realised that there was some lady who they did not know and she seems to be handling whatever ... This was the problem with big hospitals they would really look down upon you, unless you really prove yourself as somebody who can be recognised.

Mohlamme became a matron at the hospital and, like Tenza, spent decades there. Both presented themselves as proudly and specifically Baragwanath nurses. Although the group identity was not automatically acquired, it was something that, when obtained, lasted a lifetime. Annah Montso explained that Baragwanath nurses were '... still a team even now after retirement. We still meet and come together, we have a senior club which meets once a month, I enjoyed it.' The senior clubs, sometimes called 'retired nurses clubs', seem to be important meeting places for retired nurses but despite the inclusive name the clubs, which meet at various churches around Soweto, are open only to retired Baragwanath nurses. At the meetings they would, as Annah explained, 'get people to come and tell us about tax and people who work at the revenue offices ... We go out to entertainment, we celebrate mothers' day and we celebrate year ending, and we find a venue and one gives a speech or whatever. Also when one of us passes on we have to be part and parcel of that. We form a memorial service and support the family and so on.'

These groups served as social gatherings, support groups, and places of continued education. They also reinforced the idea that being a Baragwanath nurse was not simply a job but part of one's identity that remained with the nurse even after she was no longer in the active employ of the hospital.

Challenging identities: Nurses' strikes and demonstrations

Many Baragwanath nurses felt that the hospital's distinctiveness created a particular group identity. However, this identity and the nurses' place in the broader nursing sisterhood were often challenged by competing loyalties to outside political organisations and by the realities of nursing in apartheid South Africa.

At Baragwanath Hospital power lay in the hands of the white, mostly male administration and the predominantly white, male doctors. Yet the nurses, predominantly black women, were the backbone of the hospital. This reality gave them some power should they choose to withdraw their labour in protest. Yet at the same time this was a group of women who belonged to a profession that frowned upon such action. This left them in a somewhat ambiguous position. Between 1948 and 1990 three events occurred at Baragwanath that highlight the competing loyalties nurses faced.

In July 1949, amid increasing unrest at medical and educational institutions around the country, a strike occurred at Baragwanath. This strike, like others at that time, had its roots in mostly local, domestic grievances. The confrontation between the white nursing administration (backed by the broader hospital administration) and black staff and student nurses centred on measures taken to end the loss of cutlery from the staff kitchen. Black nurses saw these measures as an insult and refused to return to work until their grievances had been addressed. During the ensuing discussions both sides appealed to stereotypical identites to strengthen their arguments. The black staff and student nurses complained that the actions of the administration were derogatory 'to their dignity as trained nurses'.[43] The administration used an appeal to the same set of values to urge the nurses to suspend their action. The chief matron of the Johannesburg Hospital, under whose authority Baragwanath fell during this period, 'expressed her surprise that persons who had undertaken training for the high calling of a nurse, should be prepared to desert their patients, for the sake of a few domestic grievances'.[44]

McLarty, who was often sympathetic to the needs of black nurses and spent much of her career fighting for their professional rights, was said to have 'dealt firmly with the situation'.[45] Staff nurses were informed that those who did not return to their duties were in danger of having their certificates of registration cancelled, thus risking their ability to continue practising as nurses. Student nurses were threatened in a similar way. The severity of the threat led to the collapse of the strike, and the nurses returned to their duties with their grievances still outstanding. Perhaps McLarty's response in quelling the action could have been motivated by her desire to instil in her nurses what she saw as the correct 'professional' ethos rather than out of a disregard for their rights.

Black nurses and the white nursing administration both appealed to the same image of the nurse as a dignified professional – for different ends, and there was a significant power differential. Throughout this event power lay in the hands of the white administration, which as Mashaba, among others, has pointed out, often lacked cross-cultural understanding and often had little appreciation of the issues black nurses faced or how they felt.[46]

The late 1940s and 1950s saw the increasing politicisation of African society. Nurses who had not, in previous decades, been involved in politics began to be organised politically.[47] This heightened politicisation came at a time when apartheid was formally entering the nursing profession. The Nursing Act No. 45 of 1944 was altered by the Nursing Amendment Act No. 69 of 1957, which introduced racial segregation into nursing legislation, empowering the SANC to implement different training programmes and separate nursing registers based on race. In effect, this legislation seemed to have little effect on working practices that were already *de facto* segregated. Certainly, none of the nurses I interviewed saw this legislation as significantly altering working practice.

There was, however, much opposition to the Act, both locally and internationally. It was as a result of this Act that South Africa was finally expelled from the International Council of Nurses. There was an almost complete boycott by black nurses of meetings called by the SANA to explain the Act. Instead a separate meeting of black nursing representatives from around the country was held in Johannesburg. Here the Act was declared a 'gross violation of human rights, a brutal and unwarranted interference in nursing affairs, a violation of nursing ethics and traditions and an expression of racial prejudice'.[48] The response of the majority of Baragwanath nurses to the legislation is difficult to gauge. However, McLarty, Baragwanath's matron, was one of the few white nursing leaders who spoke out strongly against the legislation.[49]

The following year the government used provisions in the Act to demand that student nurses submit identity numbers as part of their compulsory registration with the SANC. In order to obtain identity numbers they would have to apply for a passbook or reference book – one of the most hated tools of the apartheid government. This attempt to extend passbooks to women, particularly nurses, led to angry protests. Helen Joseph, one of the founders of the Congress of Democrats and the Federation of South African Women, remembered that 'groups of black nurses in the Transvaal were holding angry protest meetings and nurses declared: "our mothers were washerwomen and they educated us. We will go back to the washtubs but we will not carry passes".'[50]

Despite the fact that many of their leaders were either caught up in the Treason Trial or unable to organise politically owing to banning orders, the Federation of South African Women, ANC Women's League, Black Sash and black nurses decided that a peaceful demonstration and meeting with the hospital administration should be organised at Baragwanath.[51] It was an important hospital, and its size and situation in Soweto made it an ideal location. Baragwanath also gained the attention of the government and the media. The demonstration was to take place on 22 March 1958, and was the culmination of the acts of individual and group resistance by nurses at various hospitals.[52]

The hospital and security communities' response to this action is significant. The Non-European Affairs Department set up police road blocks to halt unauthorised traffic coming into the area and cancelled all buses to the hospital. Police leave was called off, and the hospital was surrounded by police armed with revolvers, stun-guns and teargas.[53] The hospital administration also made emergency preparations. Before the demonstration, unfounded rumours of the ferocious actions the women were planning circulated at the hospital[54] – in preparation, all ambulatory patients were sent home for the weekend and all women and non-essential staff were asked to stay at home.[55]

Facing the police, on the other side of the road were a few hundred 'mothers' of the nurses, 'respectable, middle-class African housewives' and a few women of other races who gathered opposite the gates of the hospital.[56] This group of women was later augmented by several Baragwanath nurses who joined them during their tea breaks.[57] It 'was a hot morning and the umbrellas were up against the sun. Perhaps the police thought the umbrellas concealed weapons. It looked a little comic from where I stood as there seemed to be more policemen than protesters.'[58] Indeed, other sources suggest that there were between 200 and 500 women at the demonstration and '400 policemen in attendance'.[59] The reasons for this kind of response from the hospital and the police are unclear. Joseph surmises that they feared a repeat of the huge demonstration that took place on 9 August 1956 when about 20 000 women marched to the Union Buildings in Pretoria.[60] It is also possible that the security apparatus used the opportunity for a show of strength to deter further action.

The demonstration was, however, peaceful. Representatives of the women, accompanied by police, were allowed to meet the superintendent, matron and principal of the nurses' training college. They presented a letter of protest against the introduction of passes to women and the introduction of differential standards of training.[61] Their protest won some concessions. Nurses would not have to produce identity numbers to gain registration and while registers remained separate, certificates did not indicate race. Syllabuses and examinations remained identical for all nurses. These victories, although small in the overall fight for equality within the nursing profession, were important. Unlike those of the 1949 strike, the nurses' concerns could not simply be dismissed by an appeal to authority. The nature of the protest had changed from domestic grievances to grievances linked to broader political struggles.

During this incident, just as in the previous strike, both sides appealed to the stereotypical ideals of nursing. For the black nurses, and those supporting them, the introduction of passes for women, especially nurses, was seen as a significant affront to their dignity. Their letter of protest referred to the act as 'a stain upon the nursing profession, so universally honoured' and reminded the officials that nursing was an 'honourable profession, where women of all races met and worked as nurses, united in their noble vocation'.[62] Searle's account of the event also appealed to the professionalism of the nurse in a completely different way. In her account of the implementation of the 1957 Act, she did not record the compromises that the strike brought about; she wrote: 'Despite some initial political agitation by persons who were not nurses, in most instances, the sound commonsense of the nurses has won the day and nurses of all races are working amicably together to solve the country's nursing needs and to build up the profession, working in terms of the law of the land'.[63] Searle put the strike action down to outside 'political agitation' and presented black and white nurses as unified in their goal to 'build up the profession'.

The varying loyalties with which nurses had to contend played out in the decades that followed. On one hand there was their heightened politicisation. On the other hand, uprisings, potential strikes and demonstrations at hospitals were dealt with harshly by the hospital administration, supported by the state. Nurses, as public servants, were liable for dismissal if they took part in political activity – including strikes.[64] Pressure also came from within the profession. Stereotypical nurses were to be selfless and put the needs of their patients first; strike action was inappropriate. Many Baragwanath nurses had internalised the ideal of the apolitical nurse, and many older nurses looked back on their early days of nursing as a more professional period: 'in those days no nurse would go out on the street and toyi-toyi,' said Margaret Mohlala. Many felt that 'nurses should not have abandoned their duty ... it was not professional'. Black nurses surveyed in the latter part of the 1980s suggested that political activism that involved strikes clashed with the very ethics underlining nursing: that of professionalism.[65]

Baragwanath nurses were, however, also part of a society that was becoming increasingly politicised. Indeed, other nurses in the survey cited above suggested that the increased political involvement of nurses brought them into a community from which they had previously been set apart by their elite status.[66] This was especially true for the younger generation of nurses who entered the profession in the 1970s.

In June 1976, Soweto became the focal point of the struggle against apartheid as its schoolchildren took to the streets to protest against the conditions in their schools and the language in which education was delivered. Nurses who worked at Baragwanath during that time focused on how difficult the period was. They worked long hours without food, there was an inability to contact relatives, travelling to and from the hospital was difficult and above all there was the fear of finding one of their children or relatives among the dead or injured. Harriet Gwebu's memories of that day:

It was stressful. I was working in the intensive care unit ... When we looked through the window on the upper floor we saw smoke going up and we just did not know what was happening until there was an announcement that the hospital was 'on red'. You know, we worked on colours and it was now an emergency. Some of us were told to come and work in casualty. We could not leave or go home and there was no transport. We were becoming extremely stressed. Every time a load of patients came in, in an ambulance, everybody rushed to look if my child was not there, if you could not identify if it was your child that was dead. Half the time we were consoling each other because some people were crying. Some people actually found their relatives and it was quite, quite difficult. We worked the whole day and the whole night, because people coming on night duty could not come on duty and we could not leave. But we had also some support and provision from every sphere. There was no nurse and no doctor then and everybody seemed to be one. Somehow tragedy tends to bring people together. I just remember that when we were very tired and we were sitting right on the floor anybody going past would ask you what do you want, there was water or tea and they would bring it ... It was a horrible time.

Some nurses suggested that 1976 also saw a major generational schism. Whereas older nurses continued to condemn protests and strike action, younger nurses supported more active ways of voicing their discontent. One older nurse, who began her training in 1955, said: 'I think the change came after '76 to be honest ... this change that we, the older nurses, cannot come to terms with happened after '76 when we realised that the youth were different ... it is a generation of different people.' Matilda Mogale expanded on this: 'The nurses of the age of twenty then, they were different people. There was a difference, these were people who said they would leave their work [to strike], irrespective of what was going on ... There was a dramatic change, people now wanted to be heard, to be seen, to be appreciated'.

It was not only nurses who saw the events of June 1976 as a turning point in nurses' conduct. In a letter, Moira Russell remembered an event from the morning of 17 June 1976:

A group of student midwives staged a demonstration in the front of the hospital outside the administration offices [presumably to show support for the youth of Soweto]. They were joined by a small number of 'agitators' from outside the hospital. What happened next was something which was deeply disturbing and totally unexpected. The matrons at Bara had been, up to that point, treated with a marked degree of deference, especially by the most junior ranks of nursing staff or staff in training. When Miss Nola van Eerde, the chief matron, came out to speak to the student group someone picked up a stone and threw it at her. This act of defiance and aggression which would have been unthinkable 24 hours previously was no doubt prompted by the group of agitators who were non-staff members, but the fact that it actually happened was indicative of the beginning of the erosion of discipline and a change of attitude towards authority in the hospital which started to permeate throughout the ranks of the nursing staff, spreading over the years to include the ancillary and domestic staff. Things were never quite the same again and I realised later that we had witnessed the beginnings of a culture of unrest which simmered continually beneath the surface, erupting from time to time.[67]

While this account of the incident, from a white doctor, is the only evidence of this event I have been able to uncover, it is significant because it points to the changing nature of protest action among the nurses during this period. The power hierarchies were being challenged in a very explicit way.

While Gwebu, cited above, spoke of the way that the traumatic event brought people together, she also noted that there were heightened racial tensions, 'I think it hit hard on the doctors, suddenly everyone who was white was an enemy and suddenly they felt very threatened. A certain doctor used to carry a gun into theatre'. Similarly, Van den Heever remembers that 'on that day, or just afterwards, when the chief matron walked into casualty the student nurses spat at her because she was white. There was this polarisation that took place suddenly in this hospital'.

Against this background a third Nursing Act, Act 50 of 1978, which gave greater power to the Nursing Association, was passed.[68] In the context of the reformist strategies of the time, and increasing external pressure on the nursing administration, the Act reversed some of the exclusionary elements of the previous Acts. This made it possible for black nurses to be elected to the SANC.[69] However, the Act contained a number of restrictions which excluded the election of the growing number of nurses who were citizens of the 'self-governing' Bantustans. The Act also made strikes illegal.

Thus while nurses were increasingly politicised and continued to be dissatisfied with low salaries and poor working conditions, there was almost a decade during which no major nursing strikes occurred.[70] During this period there was, however, increasing labour unrest at hospitals – for example the resignation of 37 radiographers at Baragwanath in 1981 and a wage strike by non-medical workers at Hillbrow Hospital the following year.[71] The early 1980s also saw food boycotts at hospitals around the country. These boycotts, some of which included nurses, also served to highlight other issues. For example, a boycott of the Baragwanath canteen, ostensibly to protest the quality of the food, was also used to call for contracts to protect staff who worked overtime.[72] By this time, although nurses were not permitted to belong to unions, the Garment and Allied Workers Union was organising among black non-medical staff at Baragwanath and was instrumental in a number of strikes.

In November 1985, 900 student nurses and 800 daily-paid workers began a massive strike at Baragwanath Hospital. Although these groups originally had different grievances they cooperated in an action that had a major impact because of its size.[73] Matilda Mogale explained the support for the strike among the student nurses:

> I think it was about broader issues. Nurses were, for a very long time, barred from joining strikes and joining these political organisations and associating themselves with those who were getting their voices heard. So when they managed it was like when you are putting your hand on a spring mattress and when you move your hand it jumps up!

The strike action crippled the hospital. Workers were said to have stormed the hospital, rampaging through the kitchens throwing prepared food on the floors and against walls and turning dustbins upside down.[74] Operating theatres, medical departments and kitchens were closed down. Many doctors left the hospital, and only emergency services were being rendered.[75] The response of the authorities was harsh and they refused to recognise the trade unions that were attempting to negotiate on the nurses' and workers' behalf. On the second day of the strike, a large majority of both the student nurses and daily-paid workers were threatened with arrest as they entered the hospital.[76] They were then dismissed and given 24 hours' notice to collect their pay.[77] Nurses were evicted from the hostel.

While the strike was in progress, the South African Defence Force (SADF), Civil Defence Organisation of Johannesburg and other volunteers from Johannesburg and Soweto were brought in to attempt to alleviate the situation.[78] A journalist, described how

> [i]n place of the young and pretty student nurses in the wards one saw khaki-uniformed members of the South African Defence Force with maroon berets. It was a contrast to see members of the army, usually on top of Casspirs and Buffels with rifles on their laps, gently pushing stretchers while others prepared food in the kitchen.[79]

In a reversal of the role the security forces played during the 1958 strike, the soldiers entered the hospital as workers. Their presence elicited mixed responses. Some nurses were surprisingly positive about the role of the SADF during this strike. One nurse, Harriet Gwebu, remembered:

> The soldiers came to work here, in about 1985. This hospital has never been that clean, ever! It was the best of times! Though of course we had one or two collapsing when they saw blood or something. It was funny for soldiers; they should be used to blood. They did things, ok like soldiers, you send them to fetch this and they would be back in no time, they would do it – they ran!

This positive attitude was not universally shared. Calls were made to the 'authorities to withdraw the army from the hospital because its presence prolongs the recovery of patients psychologically and physically as blacks respond negatively to soldiers'.[80] The use of the SADF at the hospital was seen by some broader organisations as being particularly offensive because they were 'used as scab labour to break the strike of workers demanding a living wage'.[81]

While the SADF staffed the hospital, three of the dismissed student nurses launched an urgent application in the Rand Supreme Court for an interdict to reinstate the student nurses and auxiliary workers. Mr Justice RJ Goldstone set aside the dismissal as 'invalid and ineffective' on the grounds that the complaints of the student nurses and auxiliary workers had not been fully heard.[82] On the court's suggestion, the hospital reinstated the dismissed staff. This decision came at a time when the role of the legal system in the struggle against apartheid was changing. During the 1980s, a growing public interest law movement achieved a number of minor but important victories. These included legal challenges to the influx control laws, the Group Areas Act and conscription, as well as a legal fight for the recognition of trade unions. The court case did not, however, end the incident and nine of the student nurses were made to appear before the all-white SANC disciplinary committee on charges of 'disgraceful conduct' and 'dereliction of duty'.[83] They were cautioned and discharged but the actions of the disciplinary committee allowed the nursing sector to demonstrate their control over the nurses.

This case again highlights the contradictory but central position of black nurses. They were expected to meet the ideals of the profession and to fulfil their duties to their patients. Based on this view, as Iris Roscher, SANC president, pointed out, 'disciplinary action for patient neglect was the cornerstone of professionalism among nurses worldwide'.[84] Yet, the nurses were also part of a divided nursing sisterhood and members of a community suffering discrimination. They were in a position where, as a sister tutor at Baragwanath, Mildren Adelaide Makhaya, has pointed out, 'they had no platform to air their frustration and grievances, they had no platform to air their views except at large student nurses meeting where they were single voices crying in the wilderness'.[85] Against this background, many student nurses felt that they had no option but to embark on strike action.

Even while some nurses felt that they had legitimate reasons, they also felt a sense of duty to their patients that made their decision to join the strike a difficult one. A nurse who gave evidence in mitigation of sentence at the disciplinary committee pointed out that 'the strike and in fact any other strike was a traumatic experience for nurses whose job is not only selflessness but a very difficult one'.[86] For some, like Harriet Gwebu, 'Things were very tough ... on the one hand one was worried about patients, but you also felt that in your situation no one would ever look at it or listen to what you were saying because they knew you would not go on strike, because of your oath, and because you would think: what if that was my mother lying there and there was no one to nurse her? As Shula Marks has pointed out, nurses were '... caught between their duties to their patients and the demands of the comrades, between the pressures of the community and the discipline of the Nursing Council ... by the early 1990s nurses could be threatened with death for going on strike and threatened with death for not going on strike.'[87]

The 1985 strike succeeded in raising the profile of the student nurses' complaints and allaying some of their short-term grievances. Details of the strike appeared almost daily in South African newspapers throughout the latter half of November 1985, and well into 1986, despite the fact that under the emergency regulations in place at the time journalists were prohibited from entering the area. The strike, the first of its kind since striking was made illegal for nurses in 1978, also showed that hospitals were not immune to the labour unrest spreading around the country. Indeed, in the wake of the Baragwanath strike, hospital strikes took place at four other major hospitals, and throughout the rest of the decade nurses' strikes occurred around the country.[88]

Nurses' identities – as members of a professional elite and as black women in South Africa – have been shaped by contradictory and often competing forces. Status and professionalism was important to many nurses, and in order to achieve either within the conservative, white-dominated structures of the nursing administration many nurses did not engage in strikes and actions advocating dignity and human rights for black South Africans. Engagement in such actions was portrayed by the nursing establishment and – indeed the general public – as a derelection of duties.[89] Yet for black nurses who suffered under the yoke of apartheid at hospitals such as Baragwanath, engagement in political action was an important statement.

Endnotes

1   'Black nurses in white' recalls the US title *Black Women in White: Racial Conflict and Cooperation in the Nursing Profession 1890–1950* by Darlene Clark Hine. Indiana University Press, 1989.

2   EW Petersen (1958) 'African Nurse Training – Ten Years of Progress'. *Medical Proceedings* 4:10, May, p. 327. The badge, designed by Petersen, was first presented to graduates in 1954: 'Badges on the Cover', *South African Nurses Journal*, 61:4 (April 1974), p. 7.

3   Key exceptions to the lack of writing in this area include S Marks (1994) *Divided Sisterhood: Race, Class and Gender in the South African Nursing Profession*. London: St. Martin's Press; H Sweet and A Digby (2005) 'Race, Identity and the Nursing Profession in South Africa, c. 1850–1958'. In B Mortimer and S McCann (eds) *New Directions in the History of Nursing in International Perspective*. London: Routledge; and N Senokoanyane (1995) *Their Light, Love and Life: A Black Nurse's Story*. Cape Town: Kwela.

4   Data derived from AW Simpson, cited in 'Baragwanath Turns 21' *Weekend World*, 6 May 1968; L Hebestreit (1969) 'Nursing Service and Education at Baragwanath Hospital'. *South African Medical Journal* 43:21, May, p. 673; Simpson, 'Nursing Services at the Baragwanath Hospital', p. 325; AW Simpson (1958) 'Nursing Services at the Baragwanath Hospital'. *Medical Proceedings* 4:10, May, p. 325; and I Frack (1958a) 'Guest Editorial: Baragwanath Hospital, Decennial Anniversary'. *Medical Proceedings* 4:10, May, p. 250.

5   The South African nursing hierarchy, like the British, had matrons at the highest rank, responsible for an entire section of the hospital. Sisters had responsibility for a whole ward. Nurses had specific duties or worked with specific patients within a ward.

6   Marks (1994) op. cit., p. 78. See also S Marks (1997) 'The Legacy of the History of Nursing for Post-apartheid South Africa'. In AM Rafferty, J Robinson and R Elkan (eds) *Nursing History and the Politics of Welfare.* (New York: Routledge, p. 30.

7   See for example C Searle (1965) *The History of the Development of Nursing in South Africa.* Cape Town: Struik, pp. 124–5.

8   Petersen op. cit., p. 327.

9   TG Mashaba (1995) *Rising to the Challenge of Change: A History of Black Nursing in South Africa.* Cape Town: Juta, p. 61.

10   Op. cit., p. 32.

11   M Brandel-Syrier (1971) *Reeftown Elite: A Study of Social Mobility in a Modern African Community on the Reef.* London: Routledge & Kegan Paul.

12   'Only three hundred in 5 000 selected', *Weekend World,* 6 May 1968.

13   Resha op. cit., pp. 118–20.

14   Cited in *Albertina Sisulu: Freedom Fighter,* October 1988, www.anc.org.za/ people/alberta.html [accessed 10 June 2005].

15   Senokoanyane op. cit., p. 1.

16   Data gathered from advertisements in *South African Nursing Journal,* 1966–1978 and statistics in *The Hospital and Nursing Year Book of Southern Africa,* 1966–1978.

17   Advertisement, *South African Nursing Journal,* 36:1 (January 1969): 41. Advertisement, *South African Nursing Journal,* 41:10 (October 1974): 41. Advertisement, *South African Nursing Journal,* 42:1 (January 1979): 36. Wages in real terms were calculated using the South African Consumer Price Index.

18   D du Toit (1981) *Capital and Labour in South Africa: Class Struggle in the 1970s.* London: Kegan Paul.

19   Marks (1994) op. cit., p. 173.

20   H Kuper (1965) 'Nurses', in L Kuper *An African Bourgeoisie: Race, Class, and Politics in South Africa* New Haven: Yale University Press, p. 216.

21   Mashaba op. cit., p. 50.

22   Probationary or trainee nurses at TPA hospitals wore red dresses with white pinafores.

23 Brandel-Syrier op. cit., p. 256.

24 Resha op. cit., p. 21.

25 Senokoanyane op. cit., p. 54.

26 WHP, A2197, McLarty Papers, A1. 5, Letter from WF Nzeleni, Mariazell to McLarty, 3 August 1955.

27 Bara PR Archives, Poems by Joe Tshabalala, submitted to publisher Rob Royston, 26 March 1972.

28 AP Cheater (1974) 'A Marginal Elite? African Registered Nurses in Durban, South Africa'. *African Studies* 33, p. 145.

29 WHP, A2197, McLarty Papers, A2. 11, Jane McLarty, speech to Baragwanath graduating students, January or February 1966, p. 6.

30 See, for example, Bara PR Archives, 'Baragwanath: A Place of Healing', Information Brochure (nd); L Dellatola (1977) 'Soweto's Healers'. *Panorama* February, pp. 4–9; 'Baragwanath: the People's Hospital', *Southern Africa Today* (July 1986), pp. 4–10.

31 'Baragwanath – Giant Among Hospitals' *The Star*, 1 April 1969.

32 Simpson op. cit., pp. 325–7; Petersen op. cit., pp. 327–36; Hebestreit op. cit., pp. 670–4.

33 Mashaba op. cit., p. 38.

34 Hebestreit op. cit., p. 673.

35 Ibid.

36 See for example H Sweet and A Digby (2005) 'Race, Identity and the Nursing Profession in South Africa, c. 1850–1958'. In B Mortimer and S McCann (eds) *New Directions in the History of Nursing in International Perspective*. London: Routledge, p. 113; and H Sweet (2004) '"Wanted: 16 Nurses of the Better Educated Type": Provision of Nurses to South Africa in the Late Nineteenth and Early Twentieth Centuries'. *Nursing Inquiry* 11, p. 180.

37 Petersen op. cit., p. 329.

38 Bara PR Archives, 'Baragwanath: A Place of Healing', *Information Brochure* (nd), pp. 12, 15.

39 Telephone conversation with Koos Beukes, 20 October 2003.

40 Digby and Sweet op. cit., p. 113.

41 Hebestreit op. cit., p. 672.

42 WHP, A2197, McLarty Papers, B1.4, Jane McLarty, 'Summary and Assessment: Study Course in African Culture and its Relationship to the Training of African Nurses' (c. November 1954), p. 2.

43 SAB, JHM 121, 625/48(5), KF Mills (Superintendent, Johannesburg Hospital) to the chairman and members of the Special Purposes Committee, 'Baragwanath Hospital: Disturbance among Nursing Staff', 18 July 1949.

44 Ibid.

45 See also, Marks (1994) op. cit., pp. 127, 138; Searle op. cit., pp. 278–9; 'Obituary: In Memoriam – Jane McLarty (1893–1989)'. *Nursing RSA* 4:3, March 1989, p. 8.

46 Mashaba op. cit., p. 40.

47 Marks (1994) op. cit., pp. 12, 106–12, 142.

48 TO Kentron (1958) 'Anti-Apartheid Nursing Body to Confer: Protest Against Act Growing'. *Contact: The SA News Review* June, p. 8.

49 'Obituary: Jane McLarty (1893–1989)', *Nursing RSA* 4:3, March 1989, p. 8; 'In the House of Assembly: Nursing Amendment Bill Criticised by Mrs. Ballinger', *Rand Daily Mail* 1 April 1950; Marks, *Divided Sisterhood*, p. 138.

50 H Joseph (1986) *Side by Side: The Autobiography of Helen Joseph.* London: Morrow, p. 118.

51 WHP, AD1137, Fedsaw, C.C.4.7, '1957 Bill' (nd); WHP, AD1137, Fedsaw, C.C.4.7, 'Conference of Women', 23 June 1957.

52 Kentron op. cit., p. 8; Baldwin-Ragaven et al. op. cit., p. 168; Joseph op. cit., p. 64; Marks (1994) op. cit., p. 161.

53 'Non-White Nurses Protest Against Passes' *Sunday Times*, 23 March 1958; Resha op. cit., p. 120.

54 Jarrett-Kerr op. cit., p. 70.

55 Resha op. cit., p. 120.

56 Jarrett-Kerr op. cit., p. 71. It is probable that the word 'mother' is used here not to mean the actual mothers of nurses – although that might have been the case for some women – but more generally to indicate older African women.

57 Resha op. cit., p. 120.

58 Joseph op. cit., p. 64.

59 M Cooper (1958) 'New Pattern of Protest'. *Contact: The SA News Review*, 1:5, April; 'Non-White Nurses Protest against Passes' *Sunday Times*, 23 March 1958.

60 Joseph op. cit., p. 64. See also Cooper op. cit., p. 4.

61 WHP, AD1137, Fedsaw C.C.4.5, 'To the Matron of Baragwanath Hospital and the Principal of the Training College for Non-European Nurses' (nd), pp. 1–2; Resha op. cit., p. 120; Joseph op. cit., p. 64.

62 WHP, AD1137, Fedsaw C.C.4.5, 'To the Matron of Baragwanath Hospital and the Principal of the Training College for Non-European Nurses' (nd), p. 2.

63 Searle op. cit., p. 237.

64 Jarrett-Kerr op. cit., p. 71; Marks (1994) op. cit., pp. 166–72.

65 L Rispel and M Motsei (1998) 'Nurses and Their Work – A Survey of Opinions'. *Critical Health* 24, October, p. 20.

66 Ibid.

67 Moira Russell in a letter to Simonne Horwitz, 6 April 2004.

68 L Uys (1987) 'Racism and the South African Nurse'. *Nursing RSA*, 2:11/12, November–December, p. 55.

69 Marks (1994) op. cit., p. 167.

70 'Health Workers Struggles', *Critical Health*, 15, May 1986, pp. 17–9; 'An Historical Overview of Nursing Struggles in South Africa', *Critical Health*, 24, October 1998, p. 55.

71 'Other Strikes at Other Hospitals', *Critical Health*, 15, May 1986, p. 12.

72 An Historical Overview of Nursing Struggles in South Africa. *Critical Health* 24, October 1998. Similar boycotts occurred at Coronation and Hillbrow hospitals.

73 'Baragwanath Hospital Strike 1985: Divided Interests and Joint Action'. *Critical Health* May 1986.

74 'Bara Reports False – Official' *Sowetan*, 22 November 1985; 'Hospital Chaos as Hundreds of Strikers Arrested' *Weekly Mail*, 15 November 1985.

75 'Hospital Chaos as Hundreds of Strikers Arrested' *Weekly Mail*, 15 November 1985.

76 '700 Held at Bara' *Sowetan*, 15 November 1985.

77 '900 Striking Bara Nurses Given Notice' *Business Day*, 19 November 1985.

78 'Baragwanath is Back to Normal with Outside Helpers' *The Citizen*, 18 November 1985; 'Army Calls Medics to do Duty at Bara' *Business Day*, 22 November 1985; 'Baragwanath: What was Really Achieved?' *Sowetan*, 28 November 1985.

79 'Army Takes Over Bara But It's Not the Same' *The Star*, 18 November 1985.

80 'Bara: Court Move' *Sowetan*, 19 November 1985.

81 'Troops Must Get Out' *SASPU National*, 12 December 1985, p. 10.

82 'Bara: Court Move' *Sowetan*, 19 November 1985 and 'Bara Dismissal Notice "Invalid and Ineffective"' *The Star*, 25 November 1985. The application was brought by Mardulate Tshabalala, Themba Nbobo and Macbeth Nxumalo.

83 'Comment', *Sowetan*, 28 May 1986 and 'Pardon Bara 9', *Sowetan*, 28 May 1986. The nine nurses were K Mophosho, F Morafe, MT Papo, M Mpshe, J Nbobo, PM Morodi, WH Shibambo and A Shilote.

84 Cited in 'Nurses Join Forces to Condemn 'Radical Bara Activities'' *The Citizen*, 23 May 1986.

85 Cited in 'Pardon Bara 9' *Sowetan*, 28 May 1986.

86 'Comment' *Sowetan*, 28 May 1986.

87 S Marks (1997) 'The Legacy of the History of Nursing for Post-apartheid South Africa. In AM Rafferty, J Robinson and R Elkan (eds) *Nursing History and the Politics of Welfare*. New York: Routledge, p. 34.

88 Marks (1994) op. cit., p. 203.

89 Marks makes a similar point when she suggests that 'the striking black nurses' had been portrayed, from the 1980s onwards, as the "bad nurse" in narratives which seem to weave together nineteenth century Dickensian images of "Sairey Gamp" with African rumours of nurses' cruelty': Marks (1997) op. cit., p. 29.

CHAPTER 6

Chronic contradictions
The struggle of Baragwanath in the 1980s

This cartoon appeared in *The Star* newspaper on 11 May 1988, just a few days after the high-profile, successful separation of conjoined twins Mpho and Mphonyana Mathibela at Baragwanath Hospital. The separation of the twins – a medical first for South Africa – attracted the attention of the media and the medical community, locally and internationally. At the same time, the cartoon cleverly pointed to critical issue shaping the hospital. While the twins were fighting for their lives, there was another struggle being fought at Baragwanath, a struggle by doctors, nurses and patients against massive overcrowding.

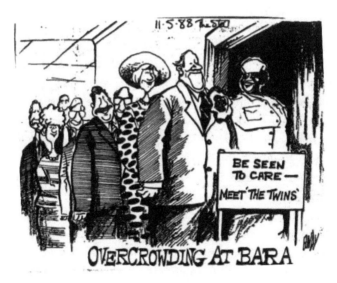

Figure 4: 'Overcrowding at Baragwanath' courtesy *The Star*

The juxtaposition of reports on these two topics – the advanced medical care available at the hospital and chronic overcrowding – highlights the central contradiction of Baragwanath's apartheid-era services. By the time this cartoon appeared in the late 1980s Baragwanath was equipped to treat an exceptional range of diseases within its seventeen specialist departments or units. Much of this growth occurred during the mid-1970s and was driven by the interests of the hospital's increasingly specialised doctors and also by necessity. For example, the Paediatric Metabolic and Nutrition Research Unit, which was opened in 1974, was funded jointly by the Transvaal Provincial Administration and the University of the Witwatersrand and carried out research into the treatment of diseases related to nutritional deficiencies in children.[1] Similarly, the Gastroenterology Unit which was established in 1975 dealt with diseases that were increasingly prominent among the urbanising Soweto population. During the next decade the unit established itself as one of the major departments of its kind on the continent.[2] The Department of Surgery had also grown dramatically by the 1980s. The original nine operating theatres had expanded to thirty to deal with the massive surgical load; between 60 and 70 per cent of surgical patients were admitted because of trauma during the 1980s and it was estimated that of the 15 000 patients admitted to the general surgery wards annually, about 4 000 were head injuries. A few of these cases were seen in the highly sophisticated neurosurgical unit that opened in the 1950s, yet a lack of resources meant that a majority of cases never received specialist care.[3]

For the Baragwanath staff, for the provincial administration under whose control the hospital fell, and for the state, the successes of these pillars of excellence (as well as the image of the hospital as technically advanced) were important. For the doctors it was a justification for their association with the hospital, and the provision of high-quality care corresponded with their role as healers. In apartheid South Africa, the provincial authorities and the state stressed the high-quality, highly technical care available at Baragwanath – their 'showpiece'. They used Baragwanth to illustrate the kind of services they were providing for the black population.

This was particularly important during the 1980s when the apartheid state was coming under increasing internal and external pressure. Internally, the rise of the United Democratic Front (UDF) and the increasing action of trade unions led to a period of intense boycotts, strikes and violence that rendered the townships 'ungovernable'. In the mid-1980s president PW Botha imposed a state of emergency, which lasted for the rest of the decade and which brought with it increasingly violent state-sponsored oppression. At the same time, limited reforms were introduced. These aimed to reinforce white control over politics while adapting certain aspects of apartheid to the changing social and economic conditions. The reforms saw the repeal of laws such as those governing the compulsory segregation of public amenities, and included an increase in state funding to black hospitals. This had almost no effect on relieving the major inequalities in the health service; but it provided evidence for the state in justifying its reforms. In this context, the image of Baragwanath as a hospital that provided high-quality care to the urban African population became increasingly important to the state.

Although pillars of excellence existed at Baragwanath, by the 1980s it was running at a bed occupancy rate of well over 100 per cent. As noted in Chapters 2 and 3, the structure of apartheid health services meant that for tertiary level hospital care the large majority of Soweto's growing population (well over a million people) as well as innumerable black patients who were referred from rural areas and smaller cities, had to rely on the 2 700 beds at Baragwanath Hospital.[4] The average intake in Baragwanath's Department of Medicine was between ten and fifteen patients a day in the mid-1950s and these numbers increased to an average intake of approximately 100 to 130 patients a day during the 1980s. In the mid-1980s there was an average of 3 000 inpatients in the Department of Medicine's wards at any given time. The daily average of patients without beds was 293. At the same time there was a bed occupancy rate of between 155 per cent and 265 per cent in the late 1980s.[5] The estimated shortfall in beds for blacks at hospitals in the Southern Transvaal region was almost 2 000 in 1988.[6]

In comparison, during the same period, Pretoria's HF Verwoerd Hospital for white patients seldom saw an occupancy rate of above 60 per cent and the Johannesburg General Hospital, also serving white patients, was rarely more than 70 per cent full.[7] White patients in Johannesburg had not only a choice of state hospitals but also a far greater choice of private hospitals and clinics. For the country more generally it has been estimated that during the mid-1980s there was one state hospital bed for every 337 black persons and one state hospital bed for every sixty-one white persons.[8]

In the early 1980s, white hospitals received a budget from the provincial authorities that translated to between R75,76 and R107,47 per patient per day, while black, Indian and coloured hospitals received between R20,54 and R40,56 per patient per day.[9] In 1980 the Johannesburg General Hospital received the upper level of about R107 per patient per day while Baragwanath received only R37.[10] For the financial year 1983/84, official statistics reported that the unit cost per patient day for Baragwanath was R46,60 (R29,78 in 1980 rands) while at the Johannesburg General Hospital the unit cost per patient day was R185,50 (R118,55 in 1980 rands).[11] By 1986/87 the cost per patient day at Baragwanath and its clinics was calculated as having risen to R140,50 (R66,90 in 1980 rands) while the Johannesburg General Hospital's figure had risen to R401,74 (R191,29 in 1980 rands).[12] These figures reveal two significant points. Firstly, the significant gap in the unit cost per patient day for black and white hospitals remained throughout the period covered by this book. Secondly, during the 1980s there was a significant increase in Baragwanath's budget and the hospital's unit cost per patient, an increase that can be explained partly as a result of the political and economic reforms, which included increased spending on black health care. The increase could also point to augmented expenditure on the specialist care which was becoming more important at hospitals such as Baragwanath from the mid-1970s. At the same time, the 'per patient' figures are probably inflated by an under-reporting of patient numbers in the official statistics. During the 1980s, Leo Schamroth (professor of Medicine at Wits and chief physician at Baragwanath for fifteen years) and the Department of Medicine repeatedly called the official patient statistics into question and showed through ward registers how the official statistics undercounted patients.[13] Faults in these statistics were also admitted by the superintendent in response to Schamroth's complaints.[14] Despite increasing funding, many of Baragwanath's wards remained under severe pressure.

The massive, almost crippling strike experienced by the hospital in the mid-1980s (in part a response to these conditions) was a manifestation of the simmering labour tensions and broader political upheavals in the country. Although popular resistance in Soweto was perhaps not as widespread as in other townships in the early 1980s, its people suffered under renewed attempts by the state to counteract the UDF. As a coordinating body for anti-apartheid organisations, the UDF grew in size and strength. At the same time, *Umkhonto we Sizwe* (MK), the military arm of the ANC, had amplified its bombing campaign against military and governmental targets. As the violence escalated, the state responded through detentions, banning, and assassinations and by stationing large numbers of troops in the township. Successive states of emergency in 1985 and 1986 saw far greater powers being placed in the hands of the security forces. Increasing reports of security force presence at and interference in Baragwanath began to surface. The level of constant overcrowding, together with a chronic lack of staff, serious underfunding and increasing pressure from the apartheid state made conditions at the hospital almost unbearable for patients and staff alike.

This chapter seeks to explore these tensions, highlighting the contradictions in the way that the hospital functioned and the image it communicated and presented to local and international audiences. The separation of the conjoined twins in the 1980s changed the way Baragwanath was viewed; the operation became an icon of the sophisticated and advanced medical specialisation which was available at Baragwanath but at the same time, the simmering issue of overcrowding was thrust into public awareness by a letter of protest, signed by 101 Baragwanath doctors, deriding the deplorable conditions at the hospital. The original letter, printed in the *South African Medical Journal* on 5 September 1987, and the subsequent fallout, highlight the horrific overcrowding, shortage of staff and substandard patient care that was the other side of services at Baragwanath during the 1980s. This dichotomy is essential to understanding the history of Baragwanath Hospital.

The Mathibela twins: Two children and a world of attention

Conjoined twins are rare, conjoined twins born alive and with a viable possibility of separation, even more so. In 1964, only twenty-six surgical separations had been attempted anywhere in the world. By the mid 1990s there had been about 200.[15] By 1980, four successful separations had been recorded in South Africa. The fourth of these, and the first to take place at Baragwanath was the separation of the twins, Nicholette and Nicholine Nthene, joined at the upper abdomen. The weaker of the two, Nicholine, who also suffered from spina bifida, died, but Nicholette survived.[16]

The conjoined twins who were destined to become possibly South Africa's most famous twins were born on 7 December 1986. They were Mpho and Mphonyana Mathibela, a pair of craniopagus conjoined twins, fused at the head, born at the small regional Tshepong Hospital in Klerksdorp. After their birth the twins and their mother Sophie were moved to Baragawanth. They soon became household names in South Africa and abroad. The plans to separate them, and their eventual successful separation in 1988, were eagerly followed by the media.

The initial discussions and investigations were not in the public purview. For months, paediatricians, neurosurgeons and radiologists from Baragwanath carried out tests and investigations. The babies had separate brains but shared some brain tissue and, importantly, had a common superior sagittal sinus, one of the major veins draining blood from the brain. Some doctors were sceptical from the outset about the outcome, concerned that the amount of money allocated for the operation and the twins' care, which cost the state approximately R1.5 million, could be better used elsewhere.[17] Dr Haroon Saloojee, who was an intern at the time, recalled:

> There were lots of other needs for children in the institution, for example spinal defects or meningoceles. There were many babies who have these defects who require treatment and the earlier you do any procedure the better the outcome ... During the time of the Mathibela twins we kept raising the issue of babies not with brains that were joined but spines that needed fixing. There was certainly very little enthusiasm for neurosurgeons to do anything serious about the problem ... That is the game we play all the time at Baragwanath, it is a resource-poor setting. So therefore to me the twins' operation was a case of the bad use of resources but glamorous.

For the superintendent at the time, and for a hospital public relation officer, the calculation was rather different. Chris and Hester van den Heever discussed it:

> *Chris van den Heever*: If the patients are here they are here. Lipschitz got his salary whether he was operating on the twins or not. Bernice Peltz (one of the anaesthetists) got her salary whether she was doping the twins or not, it was part of the job. The only thing that we got extra were a few seals, and those were lent to us.

> *Hester van den Heever*: We bought those clamps that they had to fly in – that was the most expensive thing that we had to get.

Chris van den Heever: But we used those clamps afterwards for other neurosurgical procedures.

Hester van den Heever: If you look at the cost ... it was minimal because as Chris explained everybody was still doing their jobs and getting their salaries ... They kept throwing at me questions like 'how can you allow this type of surgery to take place if you have waiting lists for other types of surgery?' You know, it is not the question. As long as we can do this surgery we can extend our teaching facilities to include training more people to do that type of operation, that is important at a teaching hospital.

These recollections point to disagreements and tensions over resource allocation and priorities that existed at the hospital at the time. However, despite such concerns, Baragwanath's chief neurosurgeon, Robert Lipschitz, was keen to undertake the operation. Lipschitz graduated from Wits in 1945 and received his Fellowship of the Royal College of Surgeons, Edinburgh, in 1950. In the mid-1950s he led a strong team of doctors, most of whom had trained in the UK, in setting up the sub-specialty of neurosurgery at Baragwanath. Lipschitz was a highly qualified, innovative neurosurgeon who had done a great deal of work on unique trauma interventions associated with stab wounds to the spine or skull. It is perhaps not surprising that he wanted to attempt the operation and was secure in his ability to do it. The ultimate decision about separation was, however, left to the twins' mother, who reportedly stated, 'You must operate, Prof, God will help you, you will see.'[18]

Once Sophie Mathibela agreed to let doctors proceed with the operation, hospital authorities turned their attention to considering how public to make the story. Historically, conjoined twins have often been the centre of public attention, whether in the fairs and freak shows of the early nineteenth century, the circuses and the 'scientific' exhibitions of later periods, or under the media spotlight when display became unacceptable. The Mathibela twins received substantial media coverage, some of which was specifically facilitated by the hospital. Key players in this were Baragwanath's public relations officers (PROs).

Baragwanath Hospital was the first of the TPA's hospitals to appoint its own PRO. The original aim of the PRO was to deal with the increasing number of local and foreign visitors to the hospital and to oversee the famous Baragwanath Choir. The first PRO was appointed in 1974. A decade later, the department had expanded to three posts and the job had expanded to dealing with internal communications through the publication of the newsletter the *Bara-meter* and aspired 'to build a positive image of Baragwanath locally and internationally, and divert the attention of critics away from the negative'.[19] A large part of the work became dealing with the media. The superintendent at the time was aware of the influence of the media; he knew that 'the press is an extremely important and very powerful organisational body ... and if you want to get on in life and you want to make sure that your hospital has a good reputation you must make peace with the press'.[20] In meeting all of these aims, the story of the twins was a gift.

In March 1987, while discussions around a media-savvy strategy were in progress, the *Bona* reporter Ike Motsapi, who had heard about 'monstrous children at Bara', approached the hospital about writing a story on the twins. The superintendent felt that *Bona*, a widely read general interest pictorial monthly magazine, would be an appropriate vehicle for the story. With the consent of Sophie Mathibela, the story was given to the magazine and was printed in June 1987 with the mother and children on the front cover.[21] Magazines aimed at the urban black market such as *Bona, Drum* and *Pace* presented material that was both didactic and aspirational, and assumed 'the combined role of primers and modern day civility manuals which offer their readers new options for individual and social conduct'.[22] In *Bona*, the story of the twins was more than a voyeuristic look at 'monstrous babies'; it was a story of progress demonstrated through the highly modern, sophisticated and medicalised process of their separation.

The story had the effect of making the twins the centre of concern for the magazine's black readers. Floods of letters began arriving at the hospital wishing the twins well, offering prayers and support.[23] Framed pictures of the twins appeared next to those of the madonna and child, and revered African leaders, at market stalls.[24]

Things had begun to change, not only for the twins but also for the hospital. A set of similarly-joined twins, the Binders, had recently been separated in a fairly successful twenty-two-hour operation at Johns Hopkins Hospital in the United States.[25] Sceptics wondered if the same could be done in South Africa and at a hospital such as Baragwanath. Lipschitz is recorded as saying: 'Most likely Baragwanath Hospital is one of the only hospitals in Africa that is capable to do such an operation and can hold its own against any other in the world. It would be unnecessary to send the twins overseas while we have the skills and a very good team of doctors here at Baragwanath, who could do the operation.'[26]

Lipschitz's words appeared in an article written by the hospital's superintendent, who had a vested interest in proving that Baragwanath was unique in its ability to perform this operation. This was the precise image the hospital administration was cultivating. Lipschitz wrote only one published article about the twins, and it makes no mention of the relationship between the hospital and the operation. Other doctors have been less convinced that it was Baragwanath as an institution that was key to the surgery taking place there. They suggest, rather, that it took place at Baragwanath because that was where Lipschitz was based and he was the driving force behind the operation.

Despite some doctors' scepticism, the hospital administration and its public relations department took up the challenge of proving that Baragwanath was a world-class hospital where such an operation could take place. At this point the media strategy seemed to step into a new phase. Rather than continuing to focus on the twins it was, as Hester van den Heever later said, 'a question of introducing the media to the medical and nursing staff who were going to be the technical side'. Lipschitz and other members of the team addressed the media at press conferences, explaining the technique they would use. The stress was on the fact that South Africa, and more specifically Baragwanath, had the expertise and the skills to carry out such an operation. Propelled by the prospect of the unusual separation the story spread far beyond the *Bona* readership and the twins became world news. The twins' progress was also followed closely by other South African publications, including the *Sowetan* and *City Press* (which had a predominantly black readership) and by the English newspapers *The Star* and *Citizen*. Interestingly, the Afrikaans language paper *Beeld* published a large number of stories on the progress of the twins. Among the international newspapers that reported on the twins were the *Washington Post, New York Times, Los Angeles Times, Toronto Star, The Times* (London), *UK Sunday Mail* and *The Herald*.

The hospital administration felt – or, at least, publicly expressed – that this effort was a success. When the last pre-operation press conference was held, the superintendent pointed out that it was 'now clear that the media were looking at us with new eyes, no sign of doubt or cynicism'.[27] When asked about this during an interview he expanded:

I think that what was important was the perception, true or false, that this was an overcrowded hospital with insufficient everything, and what ... the separation of the twins did was to show that there was another component to Bara. It marked a turning point. Up till then it was always a question of trying to defend the indefensible – after that it was a question of this is what we did with limited resources.[28]

Unlike the single-operation separation of the Binder twins, the Baragwanath team developed a unique three-step process. During the first operation on Monday 20 October 1987, the Baragwanath team began the innovative process through which they planned to separate the joined vein. A clamp was placed over the joined superior sagittal sinus. It was hoped that slow venous occlusion would occur and that the collateral veins would take over the venous drainage. The twins returned to the operating theatre two weeks later and their skulls were re-opened. This procedure revealed that the clamp had worked. However, during the initial attempt to surgically separate the veins, Mphonyana experienced significant blood loss and went into cardiac arrest, so the twins were given a few months to regain their strength before the final separation was attempted.[29]

Six months later, after they had spent their first birthday at Baragwanath and undergone a battery of tests and x-rays, the date of the final separation dawned. A week before the operation a full dress rehearsal was held. A plumber and an electrician were on standby. Wits Central Television Services were on hand to take photographs and to video the procedure.[30] The emphasis was on the fact that the operation was a medical breakthrough, and would be watched by generations of medical students to come. The filming of medical operations and the creation of medical documentaries, not least about conjoined twins, is a well-documented phenomenon that became quite prominent in the twentieth century and in which doctors were increasingly portrayed as the hero 'seen to liberate the poor twins from their physical confinement'.[31] A similar message was presented in the recording of the separation of the Mathibela twins. However, while Lipschitz is prominent in the Mathibela video, it was clearly produced as a teaching tool and thus details of the procedure, and not the story of the individual doctor, are the focus.[32]

On the day of the Mathibela twins' final operation, on 3 May 1988, the hospital's council chamber was converted into a press office and dozens of media people waited for tidings from the theatre to feed through to the world. By midday over 230 reporters had either visited or called the hospital.[33] In the hospital's chapel, a group of women from Soweto, nurses and patients, prayed with the mother. The operation began early. Gretha Drummond, the head of Plastic and Reconstructive Surgery at Baragwanath, and her team then began to cut the marked skin flaps to expose the join. The cranium was cut to allow the neurosurgeons access to the brains. Lipschitz and his team took over at 10:15 am. Despite another episode of bleeding when the jugular vein was separated, the operation was successfully completed by 5 pm and the babies were brought to a sitting position where the skin flaps were placed over the exposed skulls and sutured. The remaining area of exposed skull was covered with skin grafts from the legs.[34] Lipschitz finished the separation at 5:20 pm. The babies were finally taken from the operating table to the Intensive Care Unit. The intricate operation was completed in just over ten hours.

The news then reached those waiting at the hospital. It was over, and they were alive. Word came from one of the nurses who had prayed for the babies, 'Siyabonga Nkulunkulu, ons sê dankie, Here!' (We say thank you, God). The superintendent commented: 'Suddenly we realised, we had planned everything except for a bottle of champagne to celebrate!'[35]

The operation was hailed as a breakthrough. Both twins survived. The stronger of the two, Mpho (whose name translates as 'Gift') was able to leave hospital in November 1988 – although not unscathed. She suffered some brain damage and partial paralysis on one side of her body. Mphonyana, the smaller of the twins (and whose name means 'Little Gift'), spent months in hospital. In July 1989, she had improved enough for doctors to agree to transfer her back to Tshepong Hospital so that she could be nearer to her mother and sister. She died in 1991.

During and after the operation, the hospital made maximum use of the event. One of the PRO team commented: 'I must also be very honest with you here – we also got everything out of it that we could from our side.'[36] After the operation the PROs assisted in the publication of images by arranging for the photographs from the Wits photographic team to be made available free of charge. On other occasions the press were allowed to send one photographer to take photographs of the twins on condition that those too were free – hence the very similar images that appeared in the press.

The media seemed to appreciate this strategy, judging by the amount of coverage the twins received and the comment (in an editorial in Beeld) that: 'The successful separation of the Siamese twins was every reporter's dream – not only because it was such exceptional medical history but because of the cooperation of all involved with the media ... the friendly staff of this hospital have done their utmost to ease our work.'[37]

The separation of the twins focused a spotlight on Baragwanath and on the technically advanced medical expertise available there. The operation was portrayed not only as a success but also as one that made medical history. In a review of the first 50 years of Baragwanath's life as a civilian hospital, it was said that 'the birth of the Mathibela Siamese twins in 1986 and their subsequent successful separation will go down in Baragwanath's history as one of its greatest triumphs'.[38] A congratulatory message from the Link chain of pharmacies paid tribute to 'Professor Robert Lipschitz and his medical team on their history-making achievement which has once again placed South Africa at the forefront of world medical attention'.[39] For some of the staff, too, this was a historic event. One nurse pointed out: 'I remember that very well, I nursed them. It was one of Baragwanath's limelights, something that put us on the map more than anything before'.[40]

The spotlight on the twins focused on humanitarian as well as technical aspects. The hospital had assisted the innocent children of a single mother who was employed as a domestic worker and paid a meagre wage – a fact regularly mentioned in international media articles about the twins. The doctors had attempted to restore them to health and 'normality', liberating them from a form of imprisonment and, in doing so, serving humanitarian motives. It seems as if, in the handling of the twins, the hospital authorities were, in many ways, attuned to the shifting political currents in the country.

In the wake of the final operation and in response to the descriptions of success, a stream of high profile people visited the hospital. Mrs Elize Botha, wife of the state president, was photographed delivering personalised Northern Sotho bibles as gifts for the babies. The photograph appeared on the front page of the *Sowetan*.[41] The administrator of the Transvaal, Willem Cruywagen, and his wife; the Wits vice-chancellor, Robert Charlton: the MEC for health, Daan Kirstein; and the executive director of hospital services Dr Hennie van Wyk were all reported to have visited the twins.[42] It was not only South African or high profile visitors who were drawn to the hospital.

All of a sudden we found that we had between 2 000 and 3 000 outside visitors coming here per year to know what we are doing and to see what the hospital looked like. We also found that busloads of tourists would come in here and demand to see the hospital. We found out that overseas the touring companies put advertisements into the magazines and newspapers and they advertised Baragwanath Hospital as part of the itinerary.[43]

Hester van den Heever also recalls how two Russian reporters: '... came to visit me and to see the hospital in the 1990s. They wanted to see the hospital where the twins were separated ... and I asked how they knew about it and they said they saw the twins on TV in Moscow. A couple of years later I had the first reporter here from the New China News Agency ... and the same thing, this man said they had been able to follow the progress of the twins.'

Among the celebrities who came to the hospital were 1980s Swedish movie star Britt Ekland and the 'Bond Girl' from the 1962 James Bond movie *Dr No*, Ursula Andress. Having heard about the Mathibela twins, the actresses raised R24 000 for the hospital and the Sithole conjoined twins who were transferred to Baragwanath a few years after the Mathibela twins.[44] This was particularly significant as it was a time when few people visited South Africa owing to apartheid-era sanctions. Those who did come to the hospital found themselves at the centre of highly publicised visits, constructed so that the high profile visitors were seen as linked to the humanitarian and technical success of the operation and the hospital.

The creation and maintenance of this image of the hospital was important to the hospital itself – but also to the state. The letter of congratulations from the minister of health, Dr Willie van Niekerk, highlights this point. He wrote: Congratulations to the medical, nursing and members of Baragwanath Hospital staff on their success with the unique operation on Siamese Twins. You have demonstrated to the world that your hospital has the capability which compares with the best.[45]

As this quote suggests, the operation and the positive stories it created linked well to the government propaganda around its provision of medical services to black South Africans. Despite the fact that the apartheid regime was deeply unsympathetic to the conditions and needs of the urban African population they were keen to stave off criticism by pointing to a few success stories, such as that of the twins, to prove that they were not ignoring African health care. Stressing high profile cases such as this was far simpler than dealing with the social determinants of health.

There was also an incredible outpouring of support for the twins from various other sectors of South African society. Initial interest might have been sparked by the macabre sight of the 'monstrous children' and a voyeuristic interest in the process of their separation, yet the intensive media coverage humanised the twins. This was unusual at a time when it was more common for black patients to be dehumanised and to be blamed for their diseases. The process also took place amidst numerous references to Christianity. Sophie Mathibela trusted the twins to God. Many of the reports about the operations and the twins' lives mention the prayer services that were held at the hospital and the hymns sung as the children were taken into surgery. The Christian prayers and language were a unifying factor that added to the humanitarian aspects of the support for the twins.

The twins captured the hearts and minds not only of the Baragwanath staff but of South Africans across racial, gender and generational divides. They became household names and South Africans felt that they knew them and were in some way responsible for their future. Paediatrician Lucy Wagstaff remembers: 'I was at Bara and there was all this hype – about consultations with America and enormous expense and the people talking about the separation – and ordinary people from Soweto said to me, "You know, those twins have been here about a year have they been immunised?" I remember calling neurosurgery and they were not!'[46]

One of the founders of the Mpho and Mphonyana Mathibela Trust Fund, Maggie Nkwe said, 'The twins became celebrities overnight and they created a sense of unity in the Klerksdorp community when unity was not fashionable.'[47] Individuals and companies rallied to assist the twins and their mother. 'The support for this poor, struggling single-parent family from all sectors was wonderful to see and we were able to buy them a house in Jouberton Township.'[48]

Support from the black community was clear. For many there was a sense of pride in the technical advances that had led to the operation taking place at their hospital: 'To me it was good that something good was done in this so-called black hospital and I don't know why it should not be known in the whole world over!'[49] It is also possible that there was a sense of pride in the active participation of black health care professionals in the operation. All the nurses, including the head of the nursing team, were black and there was at least one black neurosurgeon in the team, Professor Sam Mokgokong.[50] These members of the medical team could have been seen as playing an important role in healing the twins in a modern way.

At the same time there was a strong outpouring of support for the twins from the government, partly due to the link to the way the story chimed with government propaganda. The operation highlighted the quality of medical care available to black patients at a time when hospital services were, as will be shown below, coming under extreme pressure and scrutiny. The success of the operation also seems to have created feelings of pride in South Africa across the racial spectrum – a rare uniting event.

The separation of the twins raised other important questions that deserve attention in future research, questions that include the ethical considerations in operations such as this, especially at a black hospital during the apartheid area. It was sometimes insinuated during interviews and in informal conversations with those involved with the hospital and Wits medical school that white doctors were using black patients at hospitals such as Baragwanath to experiment or practise on. There are occasional suggestions, in interviews and general discussions, that some doctors were engaged in unethical practices. One example of questionable operations that were done at Baragwanath, information about which was in the public purview, was that of leucotomies. These operations sought to treat certain psychiatric disorders by the surgical removal or interruption of certain areas or pathways in the brain. In 1975 it emerged that these operations were being carried out at Baragwanath when they had been banned elsewhere.[51] However, conclusive evidence of unethical practice has been extremely difficult to establish, and a complicating factor is distinguishing intentional unethical practice, or medical negligence, from cases in which doctors were taking short-cuts in an attempt to cope with the overwhelming pressures they faced. In the case of the twins, the issue is not that of unethical practice but, rather, whether the risks involved in the operation were properly explained and understood by the mother. It is also unclear whether Lipschitz would have performed such a risky and experimental operation on conjoined twins who happened to be white. These questions are especially complex at a time when there was a generally accepted medical belief that separation was the desired state for conjoined twins, and it is difficult to know whether Lipschitz should be praised for offering a 'normalising' opportunity to black patients or criticised for using them in his own career-advancing experiment.

Lipschitz spent his life at Baragwanath. When he was promoted to be head of Neurosurgery at Wits he refused to move to the Johannesburg Hospital, as was customary, but demanded to stay at Baragwanath. It is questionable whether this was because he wanted to stay and serve Baragwanath or whether he was driven to stay in a place where he could do specific research. The twins' operation could also, perhaps, be seen as a case where the doctor, as heroic individual, put his interests and ego above the needs of patients. Lipschitz received international acclaim for the operation and many accolades, including a gold medal from Rotary, and was also named as the Johannesburg Press Club's newsmaker of the year in 1988.[52] Lipschitz died in 1996 and left almost no writing from which to evaluate his motives. He was certainly able to champion certain projects that he saw as important at Baragwanath (he does seem to have believed in the quality of the medicine at the hospital, and was admitted there for two days when he suffered heart problems just before his death).

Finally, we must question the extent to which the separation of the twins can be seen as a success. The operation was vital to the image of the hospital as one in which highly specialised care was available. For many of the staff this was public acknowledgement of the image of the hospital they sought to portray. The public lauding of the technical sophistication of the operation, and the humanitarian nature of the care the twins received, communicated to the general public the very essence of the Baragwanath ethos. Doctors and nurses who were often criticised for the services at Baragwanath, and who were looked down on by their colleagues at white hospitals, found examples like this reassuring. These examples emphasised their professionalism, technical excellence and capability to perform operations that were on a par with those around the world. Max Price noted that 'very sophisticated neurosurgery was done at Bara and it helped raise the status and image of the hospital ... the twins' operation was an example of that'.

At the same time there were those doctors who argued that the operation was not a surgical triumph at all. One surgeon, Desmond Pantanowitz, commented, 'I personally don't think it was a big surgery triumph to separate the twins, it was just a long tedious operation.' A paediatrician, Haroon Saloojee, brought out the complexities of the argument about the operation's success:

> Then there was the whole issue of the success of the operation. I was not at Baragwanath at the time – I was at Coronation. I think while we all prayed for the babies and were hopeful for a positive outcome, certainly in my view, in terms of a medical operation the operation was a disaster. You had one baby who died and a second baby who has ended up with cerebral palsy and the consequences of that for the rest of her life. Now there were problems at the time of the operations that

were not predictable, there was blood loss, but to go on and assume that this was a great success for Baragwanath is, I think, misconstruing the facts. I understand the reputation of Bara is intimately linked, certainly in the 80s, with the success of the twins operation, but I think at a more micro level I would argue that the whole reasoning behind the operation and its outcome were in fact far from glorious for the hospital.

While there were arguments about the success of the operation, the twins were certainly celebrities in the hospital. They were cared for in a separate part of Ward 7:

> let me tell you the majority of patients did not stay like this... They were also physically separated from the rest of the hospital; they had a very different level of care. We, as residents (who often ended up seeing the majority of cases in the hospital), were not allowed in the area in case we would say something or do something which might upset the public relations apple cart.[53]

The twins had two registered nursing staff on duty for each child at all times. Before the procedures, the operating theatre was cleaned and specially painted. All this occurred amid the 'normal' chaos, overcrowding, underfunding and understaffing of Baragwanath Hospital in the 1980s.

The 101 Doctors Letter: 'Disgusting and Despicable' Conditions and a World of Attention

> It was not only positively spun stories such as the separation of the twins which gained media attention for Baragwanath. The hospital's wards were overcrowded almost from the time it opened when its 400 beds were expected to serve a rapidly growing urban black population. Although the hospital had grown to just over 2 000 beds by the early 1960s, these were insufficient to serve an estimated million-plus people living in the Soweto environs and the medical wards, which admitted the chronically ill, bore the brunt. Overcrowding hit the newspaper headlines in the early 1960s and never really left them.

During the early 1970s, Schamroth repeatedly warned about overcrowded wards, lack of staff and unhygienic conditions.[54] Conditions were made worse when the upheavals in Soweto during the 1970s brought more patients to the hospital, as a number of doctors left, fearing for their safety as the liberation struggle gained momentum. Attempts to divert patients to the newly expanded primary health clinics, staffed by nurse-clinicians, were ultimately unsuccessful. Although the clinics were a success in their own right and were often more accessible to patients, they still fed patients to the hospital. In some cases increased access to primary health care actually increased the pressure on the hospital by referring more patients to the hospital for advanced treatment. At the same time, some patients refused to use the clinics and demanded to see a 'real' doctor at the hospital.[55]

During the early 1980s, the population seeking healthcare continued to expand while the number of doctors increased slightly and the number of nurses remained static. Until the mid-1980s nurses were allocated according to bed numbers and not according to patient activity, leading to a shortage of nurses in the early part of the decade.[56] In 1986, 2 405 'other race' posts for nurses were frozen in the Transvaal – and many of these posts would have been at Baragwanath.[57] This left an average of three nurses in charge of 90 patients each night.[58] One nurse remembers that during the 1980s 'the nurses were quite stressed that they had to care for the patients sleeping on the floor. They would have to kneel down to give a bed bath under someone's bed. It stressed them to see the patients on the floor.'[59] Nurses in the operating theatres remember there being 'so many patients we were on our feet from seven to seven. It was terrible – I would not go back to that overwork! We were so short staffed.'[60] By this time the ratio of nurses to patients was 0:75 at Baragwanath, 1:66 at Pretoria's HF Verwoerd Hospital and 1:75 at the Johannesburg General Hospital.[61]

There was also a doctors shortage at Baragwanath. In 1983 it was estimated that the Department of Medicine needed seven junior doctors for each of its six medical units in order to function adequately with the large number of patients. Instead of the 42 junior doctors the department needed, the provincial administration allocated 28 junior doctors.[62] In 1985, all vacant posts, and those of doctors who left the department, were frozen, leading to a reduction of nine posts.[63] Following protests from the Department of Medicine, which argued that 160 doctors were needed to cope with the workload, the decision was repealed and the nine posts were unfrozen, giving the department a total of 89 posts.[64] Patients found the conditions in the wards unbearable. One wrote that she would 'prefer to be discharged from hospital due to the fact that I am obligated to sleep on the floor with no possibility of obtaining a bed. I fully realise that I am not yet well but would prefer to be discharged.'[65]

Journalist Thandeka Gqubule was admitted to Baragwanath during the 1980s and her evocative account of her time at the hospital is representative of a broader collection of accounts told by doctors and nurses and gives a rare insight into patients' points of view. Having arrived by ambulance, Gqubule was examined relatively quickly, but thoroughly. The examination was watched by three nurses, other patients, and anyone else in the wards. This led her to comment that 'privacy was not a priority here'. She was eventually admitted and taken, 'by a drunk middle-aged man – who had brought me a grubby hospital gown – to another ward, he wore a brown suit and I could not work out what his job was'. Gqubule described the wards she was taken to as consisting of 'three floors': a 'top floor' that consisted of closely packed rows of beds; a 'ground floor' that consisted of two rows of mattresses beneath the beds; and then the 'basement', spaces on thin rubber mats on the floor between the mattresses. It was not only the sleeping arrangements that were inadequate. Gqubule noted that in her ward 60 patients had to share four toilets and because there were no baths the patients had to wash in six basins. These conditions led her to comment that 'not even during my four-month detention at Diepkloof prison had I felt so uncomfortable'.[66]

Conditions in the overcrowded and underresourced wards made it difficult for the nursing staff to carry out their duties. There were only two nurses on duty in the ward during the night Gqubule spent at Baragwanath. Unable to cope with the number of patients, they simply could not provide the necessary care. They often found it impossible to administer medication to patients who got 'lost' or whose medical records could not be found. Throughout this period the provincial administration publicly expressed scepticism about the actual patient numbers. Where they did acknowledge overcrowding they blamed this on the medical staff's lack of work ethic and their admission of unnecessary cases. The administration repeatedly hinted that doctors were unnecessarily admitting patients to the wards and keeping patients in hospital longer than necessary.[67]

To counter this scepticism, Schamroth, who was by then an internationally renowned cardiologist, wrote regular letters to the hospital and provincial authorities recording intake numbers and what he described as the 'desperate situation' in the medical wards. He showed that the doctor/patient ratio meant that medical examinations that should have taken at least an hour to perform were reduced to a perfunctory ten minutes.[68] In another example he was able to show that junior doctors were compelled to admit more than twenty cases on an intake day and were dealing with more than forty cases a day. These numbers placed the doctors under massive stress and made it impossible to provide adequate care.[69] During the 1980s further cuts were threatened and in 1985 Schamroth warned: 'The Department of Medicine has never had a greater workload than at the moment and a reduction of a further nine posts, as the department is forcing us to make, would compromise patient care to the point of collapse.'[70] He also showed that, contrary to the belief of the provincial administration and, indeed, the hospital's senior administration, the doctors were using increasingly strict criteria to admit patients and were often forced to discharge them early in order to make room for others.

Schamroth's famous 'voluminous correspondence' with the hospital authorities and provincial administration is, perhaps, the fullest account of conditions at the hospital, especially during the first part of the decade.[71] He was determined to demonstrate that the inaction of the administration – rather than inadequate commitment and service by the medical staff – was responsible for the hospital's problems. While many of Schamroth's letters did not result in direct action, they were certainly a thorn in the side of the provincial and hospital administration and a constant reminder of what was going on in the wards. The hospital administration seemed concerned that Schamroth would embarrass them and the hospital by speaking out. For example, Schamroth's comments on the conditions at the hospital during a meeting with the TPA incurred the wrath of Beukes, superintendent at the time. Schamroth claimed that Beukes then accosted him in the doctors' dining room complaining that Schamroth, having embarrassed Beukes in front of provincial officials, had brought the hospital into disrepute.[72] In all these cases Schamroth's letters and complaints cut at the very heart of the image that the administrators were trying to portray.

Schamroth was one of the most outspoken of the doctors who called on the administration to address overcrowding, understaffing and severe underfunding at the hospital; but he was certainly not alone. In the early 1980s, doctors launched a number of campaigns to goad the administration into action. These included a delegation of registrars visiting the director of hospital Services in Pretoria to call for a solution to the suffering of patients in the awful conditions at the hospital. A delegation led by Schamroth also met the vice-chancellor of Wits in an attempt to gain the university's support.[73]

When neither of these efforts bore fruit, the doctors changed tactics and attempted to appeal to the South African Medical and Dental Council (SAMDC) which had been established in 1928 and was responsible for registering medical practitioners. The council was also responsible for regulating the conduct of health care professionals and maintaining the standards of practice and training. It was hoped that either on ethical grounds or on the basis of the substandard conditions for training, the council might react.[74] Seventy doctors signed the letter of petition addressed to the SAMDC. It called for an investigation into 'the appalling state of medical practice at Baragwanath Hospital, which we feel is in conflict with medical ethics and in fact constitutes a flagrant contravention of medical practice conditions as laid down by the South African Medical and Dental Council'.[75] The conditions included the 'catastrophic and inhumane situation where wards which contain 40 beds may have well over 120 patients', making proper care impossible.

The Baragwanath doctors raised their request at a meeting of the SAMDC, but it was decided that the discussion would be held over until a meeting the following year. The promised discussion never occurred. The SAMDC claimed that they were satisfied with the training of medical students, interns and specialists and that they would refer the issues of the hospital's service delivery to the director of hospital services and Wits since the issues were in their domain.[76] The majority of the council's members were appointed by the minister of health and were reluctant to speak out against the government, so it is hardly surprising that there was no further action on the part of the SAMDC. The Truth and Reconciliation Commission hearings (which started in 1996) pointed to a long history of inaction in the face of gross inequality and human rights abuses on the part of SAMDC.[77] While the doctors appealed to the SAMDC, a public statement by the director of hospital services suggested once again that the figures for overcrowding cited by the petition's authors were considerably exaggerated and did not reflect the factual situation at the hospital. However, he admitted that on occasion the medical wards were overcrowded.[78] The lack of satisfactory action from the authorities meant that doctors continued their campaign. In 1983, staff in the medical wards threatened to make information about the conditions at the hospital available to the media, medical associations around the world and to the International Red Cross.[79]

In the mid-1980s, senior Baragwanath physicians David Blumsohn, Ken Huddle, Louis (Leib) Krut and George Marinopolus met to decide on a course of action which might at last bring some relief to the patients and staff at the hospital. They decided to write a letter of protest that would be submitted to the *South African Medical Journal (SAMJ)* for publication.[80] The letter was drafted by Blumsohn and modified by others. Legal counsel was sought as to the implications of involving others, especially junior staff, in the letter and it was decided, despite some reservations, that all doctors in the department would be given the opportunity to sign. A hundred and one doctors, almost the entire Baragwanath Department of Medicine, signed the letter, which appeared in the *SAMJ* in September 1987.[81] The letter, and the responses to it, caused an enormous outcry and catapulted the situation at Baragwanath into the public eye and into the courts. Schamroth explained that by 1987 the situation '... has reached a critical stage. Doctors are not coping even though they work an average of 90 hours a week. Basic medical care has broken down and morale is totally destroyed. These are dedicated doctors but there is no more they can do. It is physically impossible for them to divide themselves into greater numbers. Their frustration is entirely justified and in my opinion so was the letter sent to the *SAMJ*.'[82]

In the letter, the doctors repeated criticisms that had been made in the early 1980s, deploring the 'disgusting and despicable' conditions of the medical wards. The letter further accused the TPA of indifference to the problems faced by staff at Baragwanath and their callous disregard for the patients, whom the TPA suggested were often admitted unnecessarily. The letter asserts that 'the attitude of the responsible authorities can only be described as deplorable. The state of affairs is inhumane.'[83] The letter goes on to criticise the authorities for their lack of action and to suggest that any promises to improve facilities at Baragwanath or to build a new hospital in Soweto to relieve the pressure on Baragwanath 'have proved to be devoid of truth'. The letter outlines the hypocrisy of the provincial administration's stance that there was no money for new medical facilities when an expensive administration block had been erected at the hospital in 1983 and a second R300 million hospital for whites was being planned in Pretoria. It is interesting to note here that while the doctors stress the fact that the provincial administration had the capital to invest in a new white hospital (a fact strongly denied by the administration) very little mention is made here, in Schamroth's letters or by the university, of the vastly differential funding hospitals received from the provincial administration.

The intent of the 101 doctors' letter, clearly stated in its conclusion, was that it would evoke enough response from the profession to bring about some action. The letter certainly caused a furore. Letters of support and reproach flowed into the *SAMJ* and a number were published in successive editions. The media picked up the story and several reports and exposés appeared in the *Sunday Times, Sowetan, Rand Daily Mail* and *Star.*

The TPA swung into action in the immediate aftermath of the letter, denying the accusations, especially those regarding their inaction and callous attitude. The administrators threatened the doctors with disciplinary action, dismissal or non-promotion if they did not sign a grovelling apology.[84] In the apology letter, drafted by the TPA and then altered by the doctors, they did not apologise for statements made about the overcrowding itself but focused on 'incorrect' and 'derogatory' statements, ranging from accusations made about the state's focus on white hospital care to comments about the authorities' attitudes towards doctors and patients at Baragwanath. Forty-nine doctors signed the letter, which was then published in the *SAMJ* in April 1988.[85]

This letter did not calm the fracas; rather it stimulated a debate about the circumstances in which the doctors made the apology. A number of letters published in the *SAMJ* and other newspapers and journals expressed concern that the apology might have been extracted under duress and that doctors were facing active victimisation and intimidation. One such letter claimed that the actions of the TPA were 'unreasonable and punitive, acts which should be stopped and rescinded'.[86] These threats probably led some doctors to sign the apology. Others signed out of a commitment to remain in the public sector and serve their patients despite the conditions. This was particularly so for black doctors as Baragwanath was one of the few places where they could work in the public sector.

Even in the face of the threats not all the doctors signed the apology. A group of senior doctors, mostly consultants and medical officers, submitted a signed letter to Hennie van Wyk, director of hospital services in the TPA, which they agreed on the need for both sides to contribute constructively in moving forward. However, they refused to recant while the core issue of overcrowding and terrible patient conditions had not been addressed. These doctors then received an official reprimand. They were warned that the TPA had considered 'formal disciplinary action' against them in terms of the Public Service Act of 1984 but that it was decided that they would not be fired or face any further sanction. They were, however, told that any repeat of such conduct would be viewed in a serious light. The letters of reprimand also stressed the provincial administration's disappointment in the doctors' actions.[87]

The majority of senior doctors emerged from the affair unscathed. The one exception was Ken Huddle, whose appointment as head of the Department of Medicine at Baragwanath was to have come into effect towards the end of 1987. The University supported his application, but the TPA rejected it. It was widely suspected that this was a result of his record of protest for better conditions at the hospital culminating in his involvement in the 101 doctors' letter (Huddle was eventually appointed to the headship in 1990).[88]

A number of junior doctors faced punitive action. Beverly Traub and Hubert Hon were both refused reappointment as senior house officers while Linda Jivhuho, Zolela Ngcwabe, Gideon Grame and Mark Friedman, who were all completing periods of internship, were not appointed as house officers as was the usual practice.[89] All had signed the original letter, none had signed the apology. The way the TPA was using appointments to punish doctors was made clearer when colleagues who had signed the apology were subsequently appointed to posts they applied for.[90]

The six doctors then sought through their attorneys to have the administrator's decision reversed. When the case first came before the court in December 1987, Justice Richard Goldstone set aside the decision and demanded that the six be given the opportunity for a fair hearing with regard to their applications. The hearing was held on 30 December 1987, but Mr CC Badenhorst, acting on behalf of the administrator of the Transvaal and the director of hospital services, declared that the applicants were 'not suitable' for appointment. Feeling they had no other option, five doctors apologised. Beverly Traub, however, did not. She had held the position of senior house officer for two six-month terms and had the support and recommendation of her seniors and head of department, yet her confirmation to the same position for a third term was blocked by the TPA which considered her 'not suitable'.[91]

In the case of Traub and her colleagues, 'not suitable' had less to do with their medical qualifications than with the TPA's sense of what constituted loyalty and 'correct' behaviour. Their reaction to the letter suggests that they saw it as an affront and an act of disloyalty. The TPA's image had been tarnished and it was that image that they sought to defend – though their reactions rather than dealing with the issues behind the original letter. It would have been difficult to take disciplinary action over and above the reprimand against senior doctors for their role in the protests; junior staff could more easily be threatened. Traub was not intimidated. She maintained that she had refused to sign the apology on the grounds that 'it did not fairly and honestly reflect my state of mind and perceptions of the situation. I felt then, and I still feel, that the actual conditions of the medical wards and in the department of medicine are extremely disturbing and are not conducive to effective and proper medical care.'[92]

She again instituted legal action against the administrator of the Transvaal, the director of hospital services, the superintendent of Baragwanath Hospital and the director of personnel of the TPA.[93] The case again came before Justice Goldstone. Counsel for Traub, Mr I Mahomed, argued that the only reason his client's appointment was not confirmed was that she had identified herself with the letter to the *SAMJ*. When judgment was released on 24 August 1989, the court found that in accordance with hospital practice the doctors' applications had been forwarded to the head of the hospital departments concerned, who had submitted them with favourable recommendations to the director of hospital services for the TPA, whose function it was to make such appointments. The usual case was that the director simply confirmed the suggestions of the heads of department but this was not what occurred in the Traub case. The court decided that Traub and the other doctors had been refused appointment or reappointment due to their association with the original *SAMJ* letter and their refusal to sign the apology. The court upheld the earlier judgment of the Witwatersrand Local Division that the doctors should be given a fair hearing and should be hired because they fulfilled all the stated criteria. Traub had not only questioned a decision taken by four top officials, including the administrator of the Transvaal, but she had won.

The case is significant because it brought conditions at Baragwanath and the officials' attitude to them to the fore. One example of this is the dispute over the TPA's attitude towards patients; the allegations that the 'attitude of the responsible authorities can only be described as deplorable' and that 'pleas for help have been met by indifference and callous disregard' were among those that the authorities most vehemently denied.[94] Yet a number of articles and statements made by TPA officials seemed to be based on racial thinking and stereotyping and seem to support the doctors' claims. Officials attempted to lay the blame for the hospital's conditions at the feet of the patients. They were quoted as claiming that the reason for overcrowding at Baragwanath was that 'blacks like being in hospital'.[95] Another article quotes the TPA claiming that the overcrowding was a result of the fact that 'they breed too much'.[96] In May 1987, Dr D Kritzinger, deputy director of inspections of the TPA, was reported to have made the explosive statement that 'the population of Soweto consisted of Third World people who slept on the floor at home and didn't need beds in hospital. It was official policy not to improve facilities at "Bara" until blacks contributed more to the economy'.[97] While this was never openly stated 'official' policy (from anyone other than Kritzinger), these comments certainly go some way towards showing the kinds of attitudes that existed among the provincial health authorities.

The public stance of the government was very different. The line was that improvements were being made and that more would be done as soon as the money was available. This was in keeping with government policy at the time. With the coming to power of PW Botha in the late 1970s, the focus shifted to a 'total strategy' and attempts to win support from African elites. Many of the 'petty' apartheid laws were repealed and some increases in funding to services such as health care were made. It was believed that such a strategy would reduce the opposition of revolutionary liberation movements.[98]

The TPA did spend more than R23 million on Baragwanath during the 1980s. Among the projects undertaken was the building of a new administration block that did nothing to ease the overcrowding but, rather, further removed the hospital administration from the rest of the institution by insulating it in a multistorey building. Similarly, the construction of a new R8 million nurses' home and training centre, the building of new gateposts and the installation of new boilers and a telephone exchange were some of the developments made by the TPA, but none of these projects addressed the central concerns of the staff and patients.[99] The period from the mid-1970s also saw the growth of a number of medical specialties at the hospital, some of them funded in part by the TPA. This expenditure was aligned with attempts to insure that the hospital offered the possibility of highly technical medical training for the students who passed through it and so that it maintained the appearance of a modern academic hospital; and it reflected broader patterns of health care at the time, focusing on advanced, technical hospital medicine rather than primary health care.

The 101 doctors' letter also brought Wits into the debate in an active way at last. There had been constant appeals to the university to intervene at Baragwanath during the early 1980s, but it was only after the publication of the letter that Wits took action that ultimately produced material benefits for the hospital. This took place against a background of heightened student political activism, especially among Wits' medical students during the late 1980s.[100] A number of Wits students and faculty members were involved in other medico-ethical, political campaigns such as that calling for an investigation into the brutal death of the black consciousness leader Steve Biko who died at the hands of the security police in 1978.[101] This created an atmosphere of heightened political awareness that could have been another contributing factor in Wits becoming more actively involved.

In direct response to the furore around the 101 doctors' letter, the university set up a commission of inquiry under the leadership of Professor DJ du Plessis, former Wits vice-chancellor and former head of the Department of Surgery at Baragwanath. The commission had a rather limited remit – it was to investigate the effect of conditions in the medical wards on teaching and research, and to propose solutions. The commission's report, issued late in 1988, confirmed many of the claims made in the original letter about inadequate facilities at the hospital. The report stated that 'the degree of congestion and human activity was considerable ... the toilets could be smelled from some distance away ... the noise level was unacceptably high ... preparations were being made to accommodate patients for whom there were no beds by placing mattresses under the beds.

Many doctors and nurses tried to provide optimum care amid appalling conditions, but the conditions had a negative effect on staff morale. The report also concluded that the heavy workload and congestion on the wards made teaching and research almost impossible, and it disputed the TPA's claim that patients were admitted unnecessarily, finding instead that most patients admitted were seriously ill and needed a high level of care, and that they were kept in hospital no longer than necessary.[102]

Unlike any of the previous letters of complaint, the report made a number of suggestions. It recommended increasing the number of doctors and nurses employed at the hospital as well as the urgent provision of more beds and facilities for patients. It suggested that this could be done through the reopening of closed wards, the construction of temporary wards and the use of empty beds at 'white' hospitals in Johannesburg. The last of these was a suggestion that had often been mooted by clinical staff and just as regularly refused, often without discussion, by the TPA administrators. With regard to research and teaching, the report suggested encouraging closer associations between departments at Baragwanath and their sister units at other hospitals, as this would improve teaching, stimulate research and help improve morale. It also called on the national health authorities to make public its long-term plans for providing health care in Soweto.[103]

In the longer term, the report recommended building another hospital to serve the people of Soweto. This was not a new idea – there had been ongoing discussions about the construction of a new hospital with 1 000 beds near the New Canada railway station, north of Orlando East (also in Soweto). The building of this hospital was originally mentioned in 1976, but it fell off the agenda during the period after the Soweto uprisings when the focus shifted to the construction of the primary health clinics. The idea of the New Canada Hospital was again raised during the discussions about overcrowding in the late 1980s, but no realistic plans for this hospital were ever seen.[104]

While the university's medical facility accepted most of the recommendations of the commission, the TPA was more guarded, promising to cooperate as long as the suggestions coincided with the commission's original terms of reference. The TPA agreed with the need for an additional hospital in Soweto and to the development of a long-term hospital plan, although, yet again, no details or timelines were given. The major recommendations for the immediate increase in accommodation at Baragwanath were rejected by the TPA, which said that it could not afford to relieve the overcrowding. It also refused to open 'white' hospitals to all races.[105]

What was achieved by the involvement of the university? On one level the Wits Medical Faculty accepted most of the findings and recommendations of the commission, thereby endorsing most of the doctors' original criticisms, albeit more moderately. Wits's engagement also brought some material benefits in the wake of the unproductive response to the commission by other authorities. A press statement from the Wits Medical Faculty outlined the university's plan to raise R3.9 million from private sources such as Anglo American/de Beers, Barlow Rand, SA Breweries and Genmin to provide an extra 325 beds at Baragwanath. Attempts would also be made to raise money to erect prefabricated structures to accommodate the overflow.[106] This was done with the support of the Soweto community and the Transvaal administrator, Danie Hough. While the TPA had not undertaken any such initiatives themselves they seemed happy to support those of the university and to take advantage of the opportunities this created – not only to ease the overcrowding in the wards but also to provide some positive publicity.[107] In November 1989, the twelve ward extensions built with the money generously donated by private enterprise were opened.

In other ways the actions of the university did not go far enough. The establishment of a commission with a rather limited remit might be understandable given the university's link to the hospital, yet there was also an argument for the university taking a stronger moral and political stance in the face of the conditions at the hospital and the harsh response to the 101 doctors' letter. It could for example, have refused to fill positions held jointly by Wits and the TPA when the chosen candidates were blocked by the provincial administration for seemingly political reasons.[108]

The nature of apartheid medicine: The central contradictions at Baragwanath Hospital

In the byline that accompanied the cartoon that opened the chapter the cartoonist asked: 'Where were these powerful people when Baragwanath really needed them?' While the good intentions of the well-publicised flow of important visitors expressing their concern and sympathy for the Mathibela twins and their mother were not necessarily being challenged, the question posed by the cartoon is an important one. The hospital was a place capable of specialised and dedicated medical services, as the case of the Mathibela twins shows. At the same time, it was also a hospital in which the daily functioning of medical services was grossly hampered by chronic overcrowding and a serious shortage of facilities. While government officials, provincial administrators and a host of other important people showed concern for the twins, they were quick to spring into action against doctors who spoke out about the conditions at the hospital. Yet little was done by the provincial administration to improve conditions at the hospital.

The responses to both issues, although seemingly very different, were rooted in a similar set of images perpetuated by different interest groups. In both cases it was the image of the hospital as a modern technologically advanced academic hospital that was the 'show-piece' of the TPA that played an important role in driving the response.

The case of the Mathibela twins raised the sympathy of the public, and the twins were the focus of media attention, which inspired generous donations although these had dried up by the time Mpho turned thirteen (perhaps some of the companies were motivated by the free advertising they received early on). The country was swept up in a whirlwind of sympathy based on the immediacy of the situation but which was not deep and long-lasting.

Yet the story of the twins was also important for the image of the hospital because it brought fame and renown, partly as a result of the superb way in which the media (including the black press) were brought into the case and the way the image of the hospital was managed. It was very clear that the babies got the finest treatment; neither they nor their mother were placed into overcrowded wards. The individual attention they received had an effect on the quality of their care and the way conditions at the hospital were viewed. At the same time, the technical detail that became a focus of many of the media reports about the twins reinforced the point about the technical capabilities of the hospital staff. The hospital was 'managing its image', presenting itself as a hospital where good quality, highly technical medical care was provided to the African population, and there seems to have been a real feeling of fondness that developed between the hospital staff and the twins who were affectionately called 'Ons Tweeling' (our twins).

The case of the Mathibela twins was also used by the state and provincial administration to tell a story about medical progress, technical excellence and South African ability. The state – often in the guise of the provincial authorities – was asked to demonstrate its concern and interest (albeit in a paternalistic way), for black health and medical care. The interest in the case by government officials and its coverage in government publications also suggests that it was being used by the state to highlight the high-quality medical services provided for black patients. Baragwanath, as a state-run hospital, was a key institution in the apartheid machinery and events like this could be used to highlight the 'separate but equal' strategy of the government. It was what officialdom saw as an attack on its image and the image of the hospital that precipitated the response to the 101 doctors' letter. The attempt to protect image through threats and punitive action backfired, for once this became public it fuelled criticism of the authorities. The letter was significant in that it brought to light not only the horrific conditions faced by patients in the wards at Baragwanath but also the power structures and attitudes that were preventing improvements.

In discussions over the 101 doctors' letter, the hospital administration seemed rather quiet, sandwiched between their bosses and their staff, who were at loggerheads, at a time when the hospital management was moving far beyond the provincial authorities' understanding in response to the rapidly changing political tides in the country. Unlike the provincial administration, the hospital administration was in the hands of people who, although of varying political persuasion, were in Soweto on a daily basis and had far greater contact with the community they served.

These two cases highlight the irony of care at Baragwanath. The separation of the twins is an example of the provision of sophisticated technological care in some areas when basic care was very often lacking in others. Speaking in 2004, David Seftel angrily expanded on this contradiction:

> I found it morally and ethically objectionable that you could have an environment where the majority of patients were denied basic medical care and then you had these kinds of pillars of excellence which were developed exclusively to facilitate personal professional research orientations on behalf of the individual surgeon or medical doctor who was building a reputation on the backs of unsuspecting patients.

David Blumsohn made a similar point in more measured tones:

> ... what I was saying about the high-specialisation, super-specialists ... it is great to be able to do these things, but you are running before you can walk. If the patients you have are interesting patients, you have conjoined twins, interesting cardiac lesions, interesting somethings, they'll get good treatment, but the simple basic poverty-stricken patient and the hypertensive patients they don't get good treatment.

This contradiction, one of the central themes in the history of Baragwanath and in apartheid medicine more generally, is made vivid by comparing the case of the twins and the 101 doctors' letter. The two cases are thus two sides of the same coin and represent the contradiction at the heart of apartheid medicine – the very real material benefits of western biomedicine and the difficulties that a majority of the population had in accessing these benefits. Put another way, '[d]octors say that the technology and life saving functions at Baragwanath are superb, but overcrowding severely compromises follow-up care'.[109] At the same time these cases highlight the complex relationship between the apartheid state and Baragwanath Hospital. Baragwanath doctors were able to champion causes and offer technically sophisticated services even within the apartheid state. Yet in order to understand the complex, multifaceted nature of apartheid health care, these examples have to be contrasted with the numerous ways in which apartheid penetrated the health care system for the majority of urban Africans.

Endnotes

1   Bara PR Archives, 'Baragwanath Hospital, General Information' (c. 1981), p. 7; *Baragwanath Hospital Yearbook 1992/3,* 3 Johannesburg, 1993, p. 27.

2   I Segal, ARP Walker and D Parekh, 'Gastroenterology', in K Huddle and A Dubb, *Baragwanath Hospital, 50 Years: A Medical Miscellany* Johannesburg, 1994, p. 17.

3   B Rabinowitz and D Demetriades, 'Resuscitation', in Pantanowitz (ed.), *Modern Surgery,* p. 3.

4   C de Beer, *The South African Disease: Apartheid Health and Health Services* Johannesburg 1984, p. 37.

5   DMF, Letter from A Dubb, Acting Head of Department of Medicine to G Louw, Deputy Superintendent Baragwanath Hospital, 7 July 1987.

6   C de Beer, *How Many Beds Does Baragwanath Hospital Need?* July 1988, p. 4.

7   'Apartheid Health–A Disease', *New Nation,* 12 August 1986, p. 9.

8   Anderson and Mark, 'Apartheid Health', p. 678.

9   Ibid.

10   De Beer, *The South African Disease,* p. 37. Other authors have suggested slightly different figures with Baragwanath receiving R45 and the Johannesburg General Hospital receiving R136 per patient per day for the period of 1983–1984: SR Benatar and RE Kirsch, 'Baragwanath – a Hospital in Despair', *South African Medical Journal,* 72 September 1987, p. 307. While the exact figures vary slightly, the ratio remains similar and spending was clearly vastly unequal.

11   *Hospital and Nursing Year Book of Southern Africa* Cape Town, 1985, p. 161.

12   *Hospital and Nursing Year Book of Southern Africa* Cape Town, 1988, p. 264.

13   See, for example, DMF, Schamroth to Van den Heever pointing out problems in the ward statistics, 2 August 1983; Schamroth to Van den Heever shows that official statistics were incorrect, 8 November 1983; Schamroth to Sister

MI O'Mahoney (Chief Matron) on inaccurate ward numbers provided by the administration, 8 November 1983.

14 DMF, Van den Heever to Schamroth, 'Midnight Return Statistics', 20 July 1984.

15 AD Dreger, 'The Limits of Individuality: Ritual and Sacrifice in the Lives and Medical Treatment of Conjoined Twins', *Studies in the History and Philosophy of Biology and Biomedical Science*, 29, 1988, p. 5.

16 S Levin, 'Siamese Twins: Double Trouble', *Nursing RSA*, 4:7, July 1989, p. 14.

17 Legislature Documents, Replies to Written Questions, Pretoria–Witwatersrand–Vereeniging Provincial Legislature, No 70 – 1994: First Session, First Legislature (5 December 1994), p. 203, section 1 (b).

18 VdH Papers, C van den Heever, 'Ons Tweeling' (unpublished paper, July 1988); Bara PR Archive, *Barameter*, July 1988, p. 4.

19 'Department of Public Relations: Building a Positive Image', *Baragwanath Hospital Yearbook 1992/3*, 3, Johannesburg, 1993, pp. 80–3.

20 C van den Heever, 6 October 2004.

21 I Motsapi, 'These Babies are a Gift from God, says Mother', *Bona*, June 1987, pp. 59–61.

22 S Laden, 'Who's Afraid of the Black Bourgeoisie? Consumer Magazines for Black South Africans as an Apparatus of Change', *Journal of Consumer Culture*, 3, 2003, p. 197.

23 Bara PR Archive, *Barameter*, July 1988, p. 4.

24 My thanks to Professor David Coplan for alerting me to these pictures.

25 G Drummond, P Scott, D Mackay and R Lipschitz, 'Separation of the Baragwanath Craniopagus Twins', *British Journal of Plastic Surgery*, 44:1, January 1991, p. 49.

26 C van den Heever, 'New Hope for Siamese Twins', *Transhosp Nuus/News*, 4:1, December 1987, p. 1.

27 VdH Papers, C van den Heever, 'Ons Tweeling' (unpublished paper, July 1988), p. 3. See also Bara PR Archive, *Barameter*, July 1988, p. 4.

28 C van den Heever, 6 October 2004.

29 WHSL, 'The Medical Record of the Separation of the Mathibela Siamese Twins' [video recording], Johannesburg, 1988.

30 WHSL, 'The Medical Record of the Separation of the Mathibela Siamese Twins' [video recording], Johannesburg, 1988. See also, 'Bara's Twins', *Baragwanath Hospital Yearbook 1992/3*, 3, Johannesburg, 1993, pp. 80–3.

31 Van Dijck, 'Medical Documentary', pp. 541–2.

32   WHSL, 'The Medical Record of the Separation of the Mathibela Siamese Twins' [video recording], Johannesburg, 1988.

33   Bara PR Archives, 'Media Book–April–June 1988'.

34   Drummond, Scott, Mackay and Lipschitz, 'Separation of the Baragwanath Craniopagus Twins', pp. 50–1.

35   VdH Papers, C van den Heever, 'Ons Tweeling' (unpublished paper, July 1988), p. 5.

36   Hester van den Heever, 6 October 2004.

37   'Department of Public Relations', pp. 80–3.

38   'Bara's Twins', p. 80.

39   Bara PR Archive, *Barameter*, July 1988, p. 3.

40   Harriet Gwebu, 16 August 2003.

41   'Elize Botha Visits Twins', *Sowetan*, 11 May 1988.

42   Bara PR Archive, *Barameter*, July 1988, p. 2; SAB, Foto 19862, 'Mr WA Cruywagen, Administrator of Transvaal, and Mrs S Cruywagen during their visit to the Siamese twins born in the Baragwanath Hospital' (no date).

43   Hester van den Heever, 6 October 2004.

44   BHBR, Minutes of the 251st Hospital Board Meeting, 25 January 1989, p. 3; Bara PR Archive, 'Bond Girls Raise R24 000 for Bara', *Barameter*, June 1989, p. 4; T Younghusband, 'Tearful Britt holds Sithole Babies', *The Star*, 17 January 1989.

45   Bara PR Archives, 'Media Book–April–June 1988'.

46   Lucy Wagstaff, 14 September 2004.

47   Cited in C Thompson 'Famous Siamese Twin to Turn 13', *Caxton*, 1 December 1999.

48   Cited in ibid.

49   Harriet Gwebu, 16 August 2003.

50   Makhetha, 'The Matibela Siamese Twins', pp. 10–3. Mokgokong is currently Professor and Chief Neurosurgeon at Ga-Rankuwa Hospital and Medunsa. He headed the teams that separated the Makwaeba conjoined twins in 1994 and the Banda twins in 1997.

51   See, for example, T Stirling, 'Controversial Brain "Ops" Revived', *Sunday Times*, 5 January 1975; 'Black Brain Surgery Denied', *The Star*, 6 January 1975; 'Surgeon Tells of Brain Ops on Psychotics', *Rand Daily Mail*, 8 January 1975.

52   Bara PR Archive, *Barameter*, July 1988, p. 5; 'FW, 89's Newsmaker of the Year', *Die Beeld*, 10 November 1989.

53   David Seftel, 7 July 2004.

54   [zRPz]Administrator, Transvaal, and Others v. Traub and Others 1989 (4) SA 731 (A), Appendix 'G', A Letter from Schamroth to Dr HA Grove, Director of Hospital Service, 15 January 1973, p. 192, Letter from Schamroth to Dr Kniep, Superintendent of Baragwanath Hospital, 19 December 1973, p. 196 and Letter from Schamroth to Dr Beukes, Superintendent of Baragwanath Hospital, 30 July 1979, p. 199.

55   'The Steadily Rising Tide Threatens to Drown Baragwanath', *Sunday Express*, 19 June 1983; PJ Beukes, 'The Birth and First 10 Years of Primary Health Care in Soweto' (unpublished paper, August 2004), copy given to me by the author.

56   DMF, Schamroth to Van den Heever, 19 August 1985; DMF, Medical Advisory Committee, Extra Ordinary meeting, 10 May 1985, pp. 1–2.

57   Adler Museum, 'Full Report of the Du Plessis Commission', 9 August 1988, Annexure 12.1, pp. 14–9.

58   Administrator, Transvaal, and Others v. Traub and Others 1989 (4) SA 731 (A), Appendix 'G', Letter to PJ Beukes from L Schamroth, 20 August 1979, p. 202.

59   Harriet Gwebu, 16 August 2003.

60   Zodwa Mfete, 9 January 2003.

61   DMF, Medical Advisory Committee, Extra Ordinary meeting 10 May 1985, pp. 1–2.

62   DMF, Schamroth to Van den Heever, 10 January 1983. See also DMF, Schamroth to H Stein, Chairman Medical Advisory Committee, Baragwanath Hospital, 14 July 1983 and DMF, Schamroth to Grove, 27 July 1983.

63   DMF, PC Arnott, Deputy Superintendent to Schamroth, 17 December 1984; DMF Schamroth to Van den Heever, 12 February 1985.

64   DMF, Grove to Van den Heever, 11 March 1985.

65   DMF, Letter from Alina Mtshweni to Dr Mendelson, 24 March 1980.

66   T Gqubule, 'My Night Under the Bed at Bara', *Weekly Mail*, 9 December 1988.

67   'The Problem: a Racial Imbalance in Services', *Sunday Express*, 14 August 1983.

68   Administrator, Transvaal, and Others v. Traub and Others 1989 (4) SA 731 (A), Appendix 'C' Table of Statistics 'Department of Medicine, Ward

Occupancy Statistics provided by Corridor Matron Mrs Maumakwe for four Medical Wards, June 1980'; DMF, Letter from Schamroth to Arnott, 23 July 1984, p. 180.

69   DMF, Letter from Schamroth to Van den Heever, 1 July 1983; DMF, Letter from Schamroth to Van den Heever, 12 July 1983; DMF, Letter from Schamroth to Dr L Faivelsohn, Deputy Superintendent, Baragwanath Hospital, 19 July 1983.

70   DMF, Letter from Schamroth to Van den Heever, 12 February 1985.

71   These letters now form part of the DMF and thanks are due to Professor Ken Huddle for alerting me to the existence of these letters and for providing me with access to the files. Chris van den Heever, 6 October 2004 also discussed Schamroth and his correspondence.

72   DMF, Letter from Schamroth to PJ Beukes, Chief Superintendent, 22 July 1980; DMF, Beukes to Schamroth, 15 August 1980.

73   DMF, K Huddle, D Blumsohn and B Traub, 'A Proud Record of Protest', Draft Submission by the Department of Medicine, Baragwanath Hospital to the Truth and Reconciliation Commission (no date), p. 1.

74   L Baldwin-Ragaven, J de Gruchy and L London, *An Ambulance of the Wrong Colour: Health Professionals, Human Rights and Ethics in South Africa,* Cape Town, 1999, pp. 143–4.

75   DMF, Letter to the Registrar, South African Medical and Dental Council, signed by 70 Members of the Department of Medicine, Baragwanath Hospital, 12 June 1980.

76   NM Prinsloo, 'Conditions at Baragwanath Hospital', *South African Medical Journal,* 72, November 1987, p. 643.

77   Baldwin-Ragaven, De Gruchy and London, *An Ambulance of the Wrong Colour,* pp. 143–8; *Truth and Reconciliation Commission of South Africa: Final Report,* Cape Town, 1998, Vol 4, Chapter 5, p. 156.

78   'Bara-meter', *Saturday Star,* 14 October 1981.

79   DMF, Schamroth, records of meeting with Dr S Cronje S, TPA, 19 July 1983.

80   DMF, Medical Advisory Committee, Extra Ordinary Meeting, 10 May 1985, pp. 1–2.

81   'Conditions at Baragwanath Hospital', *South African Medical Journal,* 72, September 1987, p. 361.

82   Administrator, Transvaal, and Others v. Traub and Others 1989 (4) SA 731 (A), Appendix 'G', Schamroth Affidavit, p. 8.

83 'Conditions at Baragwanath Hospital', *South African Medical Journal*, 72, September 1987, p. 361.

84 Wits Archives, Bara. B2, A Byrne, 'Press Statement by the Public Relations Officer of the Transvaal Provincial Administration', 7 January 1988; DMF, Letter from Provincial Secretary to Dr K Huddle, Publication of a Letter in the *South African Medical Journal*, 5 September 1987: Baragwanath Hospital, 28 January 1988.

85 *South African Medical Journal*, 73, 2 April 1988, p. 438. See also media report MJ Woods, '49 Doctors Apologise', *Business Day*, 14 April 1988.

86 The Executive Committee of the Board of the Faculty of Medicine at Wits, 'Conditions at Baragwanath', *South African Medical Journal*, 73, 2 April 1988, p. 437.

87 DMF, Letter from Van Wyk, Publication of a Letter in the *South African Medical Journal*, 5 September 1987 – Baragwanath Hospital, 23 April 1988.

88 DMF, Van Wyk to Robert Charlton, Vice-Chancellor and Principal, Wits, 19 October 1988; DMF, K Huddle to M Marais, The Office of the Provincial Secretary, 9 November 1988.

89 DMF, Letter from Dr KD Bolton, Acting Head Department of Paediatrics Baragwanath Hospital to Van den Heever, 'Re: SHO Appointments for 1988', 29 October 1987; 'Defiant Doc puts Career on the Line for Sake of Free Speech', *Saturday Star*, 6 August 1988.

90 'Bara Dossier of Shame', *Sunday Times*, 2 October 1988.

91 DMF, Professor C Rosendorff, Faculty of Medicine, University of the Witwatersrand, 'Fact Sheet Relating to the Non-Appointment of Medical Personnel at Baragwanath Hospital', 8 December 1987; Administrator, Transvaal, and Others v. Traub and Others 1989 (4) SA 731 (A), Founding Affidavit, B Traub, p. 1–18.

92 'Defiant Doc puts Career on the Line for Sake of Free Speech', *Saturday Star*, 6 August 1988.

93 [zRPz]Administrator, Transvaal, and Others v. Traub and Others 1989 (4) SA 731 (A); A 'Judgment Reserved in Medic's Plea on Bara Decision', *The Citizen*, 30 September 1988.

94 'Conditions at Baragwanath Hospital', *South African Medical Journal*, 72, September 1987, p. 361.

95 'The Problem: A Racial Imbalance in Services', *Sunday Express*, 14 August 1983.

96   S Martin, '"They Breed too Much" was Official's Retort of Full Bara', *Sunday Star*, 2 October 1988.

97   Ibid.; 'Bara Dossier of Shame', *Sunday Times*, 2 October 1988. See also DMF, Schamroth Memorandum, 24 February 1987 which records a conversation between Kritzinger, Schamroth, Blumsohn and Krut where Kritzinger expressed similar sentiments.

98   M Swilling and M Phillips, 'State Power in the 1980s: From "Total Strategy" to Counter-Revolutionary Warfare'. In J Cock and L Nathan (eds.), *War and Society: The Militarisation of South Africa*, Cape Town, 1989, pp. 134–48.

99   Administrator, Transvaal, and Others v. Traub and Others 1989 (4) SA 731 (A), Affidavit, H van Wyk, pp. 112–3; H van Wyk, Director of Hospital Services, TPA, 'Conditions at Baragwanath', *South African Medical Journal*, 72, November 1987, p. 791; P Kramer, 'Bara One of the Best, Says Hospital Service Chief', *Sunday Express*, 10 March 1985. Chris van den Heever, 24 January 2003 also talks about developments during the 1980s.

100   Max Price, 30 August 2004; WHSR, 'Draft Submission to the Truth and Reconciliation Commission from the Faculty of Health Sciences, University of the Witwatersrand' (no date), pp. 12–3.

101   For a summary of the involvement of Wits faculty and students see J Browde, P Mokhoba and E Jassat, *University of the Witwatersrand Faculty of Health Science, Internal Reconciliation Commission Report*, Johannesburg, 1998, p. 248.

102   Wits Archives, Bara B2, Abridged Report of the Du Plessis Commission, 24 November 1988, p. 5.

103   Wits Archives, Bara, B2, Full Report of the Du Plessis Commission, 9 August 1988, pp. 14–9.

104   C van den Heever interview, 24 January 2003; R Taylor, 'Four Years On, and No Sign of New Hospital', *Rand Daily Mail*, 13 June 1980.

105   J Smith 'Baragwanath: the Squalor of Segregation', *British Medical Journal*, 298, March 1989, pp. 773–4.

106   Wits Archives, Bara. B2.4/7, Professor Clive Rosendorff, dean of the Wits Faculty of Medicine, Press Statement, 18 January 1989.

107   See for example 'Bara's Patients get Beds', *The Star*, 29 September 1989, which contains a photograph of Transvaal MEC for hospital services Daan Kirstein, standing smiling next to a patient in a new ward.

108   WHSR, IRC, Email evidence submitted by M Tikly, Head of Rheumatology, Chris Hani Baragwanath Hospital to Advocate Jules Browde, Wits IRC,

5 June 1998; DMF, K Huddle, D Blumsohn and B Traub, 'A Proud Record of Protest', Draft Submission by the Department of Medicine, Baragwanath Hospital to the Truth and Reconciliation Commission (no date), p. 4.

109 'Bara – too Many Patients, too Many Deaths', *Rand Daily* Mail, 13 April 1982.

CHAPTER 7

Baragwanath's Transition and Legacy

In 1990 South Africa entered a period of transition to democracy. President FW de Klerk announced the unbanning of the ANC, the Pan Africanist Congress and the Communist Party. Nelson Mandela and his fellow political prisoners began to be released and South Africa was on the path to its first democratic election. A new phoenix was born at Baragwanath, a phoenix that was to live through tumultuous times.

The changes in hospital policy, discussed in Chapter 1, began the process of transition. Not only was Baragwanath officially desegregated but its administration also became further centralised. This did little to affect daily functioning. The historical problems of staff shortages, lack of funding and ever-increasing patient numbers continued to plague the hospital which faced, in addition, the new challenges of HIV/AIDS, a gradual breakdown in discipline and management structures, and increasing labour tensions. The major strikes that occurred at the hospital in 1992 and 1995 set the background for Baragwanath's transition, one marked by continuity and change.

According to the *South African Medical Journal* of August 1992, the first diagnosed cases of HIV/AIDS were recorded at Baragwanath in 1987. By December 1990, 181 HIV-positive black adults had been admitted to the medical wards. Four times this number had been identified as HIV-positive. Half of these patients were in the late stages of HIV infection and two years later thirty-four per cent of those diagnosed in 1990 had died. In 1990, fifty-one symptomatic children were also identified at Baragwanath.

Over the next few years the numbers continued to grow and HIV/AIDS quickly became an important aspect of the increasing workload and the increase in in-hospital mortality. HIV-related paediatric deaths during hospital stays at Baragwanath increased from eleven children in 1992 to 111 deaths in 1996. Seeing the challenges that HIV/AIDS was posing for the hospital, even in those early years, the Department of Obstetrics and Gynaecology and that of Paediatrics at the University of the Witwatersrand developed the Baragwanath Perinatal HIV Research Unit which was initiated in 1991 by Dr James McIntyre. By 1995 the unit was formalised, and it has continued to be overseen by McIntyre and Dr Glenda Gray.

By the mid-1990s the virus was responsible for almost forty per cent of admissions to the hospital's general wards. This was just an inkling of what was to come. The full impact of the HIV/AIDS pandemic on Baragwanath Hospital was really only felt in the new millennium.

While the HIV/AIDS pandemic was beginning to gain a foothold in the hospital, Baragwanath was facing more immediate transitional upheavals. For many of Baragwanath's staff the most noteworthy event of the transition period was the 1992 strike. Karl von Holdt and Bethuel Maserumule, the only researchers to have published on this period of Baragwanath's history, suggest that the 1992 strike was an important turning point.[1] Significantly, they argue that the strike was a product of the transition rather than of the struggle against apartheid. It was only with the changes brought about during the transition that trade unions won the right to organise in the public sector and making strike action a possible method of protest.

Years later, Van den Heever noted the shift to unionisation as an important feature of the transition of the hospital:

> In 1985 with that nurses strike, these were student nurses that struck and the idea was that it was the beginning of unionisation of the nursing profession and the health care professions ... but from 1985 we saw unionisation coming in and I think a lot of hard work and effort went into the mobilisation of the Baragwanath component, from the 1980s up to the big strike of 1992.

Indeed the latter part of the 1980s saw increasing coordinated labour action among health care workers. On 27 and 28 June 1987, workers from the education, health, government and social welfare sectors launched Nehawu, the National Education Health and Allied Workers Union. The union was an affiliate of the Congress of South African Trade Unions, Cosatu. But within the oppressive conditions of apartheid South Africa its development was slow. By

1988, Nehawu had only 6 000 members nationally, drawn mostly from health sector support workers.

The health sector unions continued to gain strength into the 1990s. In 1991 a negotiated amendment to the 1988 Labour Relations Act made provision for protected strike action by employees, subject to certain conditions. While this did not specifically exclude health professionals from the right to strike it still considered strike action a breach of contract punishable by disciplinary action.

In 1992 unprecedented strike action took place among public sector health workers around the country. It was, however, protest action at Baragwanath in early June, and the response to it, that sparked mass action – by mid-1992, twenty to thirty thousand health workers across the country, mostly members of Nehawu and the Health Workers Union (HWU), were on strike. In the Transvaal alone, twenty-nine different institutions were affected and approximately 10 000 employees, mostly general assistants, participated in the strike action. Of these about 1 500 were employed at Baragwanath. The grievances dealt mainly with hospital-related issues: wages and conditions of employment. As in earlier strikes, the reaction from the TPA and from the Baragwanath Hospital management was swift and harsh. Officials warned the strikers and sent Nehawu several ultimatums demanding that they 'normalise' the situation,[2] which did little to quell the escalating violence and destruction of hospital property. During the course of the strike the TPA obtained four Supreme Court interdicts, the 'prime objective of which ... [was] to normalise the prevailing disruptive situation'.[3] When even these interdicts failed to restore order or persuade the workers to return to work, the TPA took harsher action and dismissed 7 400 workers, the bulk of them at Baragwanath Hospital. In an act which further antagonised the strikers, hospital management at Baragwanath employed large numbers of replacement workers and, in some cases, called in army medics.[4]

Despite Nehawu's call for 'total support for a strike and in a sense [sic] that we would destroy the health services',[5] most of Baragwanath's doctors and nurses did not have a sustained role in the strike, specifically because their needs were not in line with the demands of the majority of those on strike. However, in the face of increasing intimidation and with the clerks on strike and nobody to prepare their pay packets, nurses, and to a lesser extent doctors, threatened to join the strike if they were not paid.[6] Nurses also felt aggrieved that they had to fetch supplies and carry out non-medical duties which they saw as an affront to their dignity and professional status.[7]

The few nurses who did actively involve themselves in militant action during the 1992 strike were predominantly student and junior nurses. These politically active nurses were aware of the existing generational divide and reminded senior nurses that they were not immune to the discrimination of the apartheid regime: 'We call upon matrons to join us on this march because they are also BLACK OPPRESSED AND UNDERPAID.'[8] However, the hierarchical nature of the nursing profession meant that younger nurses were soon brought under the control of SANA and their more conservative seniors.[9] Even hospital management acknowledged this point; when reporting on the student nurses' actions they concluded that the opposing view of registered nurses prevailed. Nurses continued to work, even under pressure.

Another notable feature of this strike was that it was marred by intimidation and violence. Several thinly veiled death threats circulated during the strike: for example, letters which stated that the 'current industrial action ... may lead to violence and loss of life'.[10] One letter, on a Nehawu letterhead and written in Sepedi, stated:

> We also call peacefully on all nursing personnel and all others to strike. The struggle we fight will also be to your advantage. The needs that Nehawu is demanding are related to [the] ones received by workers internationally. So we are requesting all government workers to stop working so that government can listen to us. So we are giving [a] friendly warning to those who are ignoring our pleas [to strike]. If they don't support us there will be consequences. Tell your brother, sister, mother, friend, partner, neighbour, or anyone who ignores our request that their days are numbered.[11]

During the strike there were three petrol bombs in Soweto, each directed at the home of a hospital employee. In one particularly graphic case, professional nurse Lettie Mmakgang Makgotloe had her house torched by a group of over fifty individuals she considered linked to the strike.[12] A number of nurses and other non-striking workers were sjamboked and assaulted as they tried to make their way to work. Rumours that scab labourers had been shot constantly circulated at the hospital. Nehawu condemned the violence, claiming that it was not Nehawu members who were intimidating non-strikers, accusing 'agent provocateurs or the TPA for carrying out the violence',[13] and claiming that 'intimidation, assaults and arson [were] directed against strikers and strike breakers alike, particularly black nurses who continued working'.[14] In August, Nehawu marshals were deployed to monitor the situation.

After almost ten months of strikes and negotiations an agreement was signed in February 1993. The agreement regulated all aspects of the relationship between the TPA and Nehawu and served as a guide for dispute resolution, protest action and representation.[15] The strike had irreparably changed power relations within the hospital and between the hospital and the authorities. At the heart of the 1992 strike was the newly-powerful trade union Nehawu. With Nehawu's support, non-medical hospital staff began to have a voice and influence they had never held before. There were changing power structures among the medical staff too. Although the nursing hierarchy had prevailed and junior nurses were reined in, the generational divide that first developed during the mid-1970s was continuing to widen. This, and unionisation and the declining power of the SANA and SANC, meant that over the next few years the control of nursing and its disciplinary structure changed altogether.

The 1992 strike also marked a shift in the scale of Baragwanath's involvement in broader political issues. This book has shown that during the apartheid era Baragwanath served the people who were both the direct and indirect victims of the regime's harsh and oppressive rule. Conditions at the hospital were fundamentally shaped by apartheid. At the same time this book has highlighted the nuances and contradictions within this system and the subtle ways that staff at the hospital mobilised against the apartheid regime. Yet the transition period saw a much bolder and more overt engagement of the hospital and its staff in national-level politics. The 1992 strike is an important example of this.

Neal Thobejane, assistant general secretary of Nehawu, stated during a meeting with the TPA that 'although the strike is not part of the mass action of the Cosatu/ANC alliance, it slots into the programme and it cannot be divorced from mass action'.[16] Phillip Dexter, Nehawu's general secretary, linked the strike more directly to the broader political struggle. He maintained that the strike was part of 'the big political issues such as mass action' and that 'it is part of the total action to ask the Government to go'.[17] Indeed, a number of the pamphlets and posters employed at Baragwanath during the strike made reference to both hospital-related demands and to broader political issues, and while the strike might have been sparked by local issues relating to the hospital, the political climate in the country and the involvement of Nehawu did engage broader issues. As the strike progressed there was a moving away from demands on salaries and working conditions to a set of demands that became increasingly unclear but were underpinned by a call to bring about a new order.

The ashes of the strike were still smouldering when out of them was born yet another phoenix. Its birth heralded much hope. Nelson Mandela became South Africa's first black president on 10 May 1994. He appointed Dr Nkosazana Dlamini-Zuma as his first minister of health and entrusted to her the unenviable task of reforming the health care system. Central to the transition of the health care system and to transition more broadly was the Freedom Charter of 1955. This statement of principles, which the ANC had held at its core for almost five decades, called for a preventive health scheme to be run by the state; free medical care and hospitalisation for all, and 'special care for mothers and young children'. The ANC government's Reconstruction and Development Programme (RDP), adopted in 1994, also remained true to the aims of the Freedom Charter in the health care area; the focus was shifted to primary health care, especially for under-resourced provinces and rural areas. This guiding principle did not augur well for large tertiary hospitals, and especially not for Baragwanath, situated in South Africa's wealthiest province, and Baragwanath continued to buckle under huge pressure from ever-increasing patient numbers and now-decreasing resources. Not even a year later, the lack of resources led to another crippling strike, this time led by nurses.

Changes in nursing policy since the 1992 strike meant that, by 1995, nurses, for the first time since 1944, were not forced to join a predominantly white-led association. They could now legally join trade unions, and some nurses chose to join large multisector health worker unions such as Nehawu, which was affiliated with Cosatu; or the Health and Other Service Personnel Trade Union of South Africa (Hospersa), which fell under the umbrella of the Federation of Unions of South Africa (Fedusa). Many, however, preferred to form their own professional body. This is hardly surprising given nurses' backgrounds and the way in which they saw themselves as professionals who held a specific status within the hospital and society because of their training. During this time nurses formed their own national union, the South African Democratic Nurses Union (Sadnu). Sadnu refused to seek affiliation with either of the country's two major union federations, Cosatu or the National Council of Trade Unions (Nactu).

Late in 1994, in the Public Sector Bargaining Chamber, various health sector unions negotiated good increases for their nonprofessional members. These workers received an increase of over twenty per cent. By August 1995, nurses working for municipal clinics in Gauteng were receiving an increase of twelve per cent to fifteen per cent, while those working in provincial hospitals (like Baragwanath) received only five per cent – considered appropriate by the SANA and by both Nehawu and Hospersa. Nurses considered the increase degrading and totally inappropriate and continued their wildcat strikes, voicing grievances over 'shifts, grading, lack of workplace consultation and poor working conditions'.[18] They also demanded equal salaries for all local authority employees and a revised tax system for nurses. By mid-August a wage deadlock between black nurses and government had occurred, and almost 2 000 Baragwanath nurses embarked on a full-scale strike which lasted for almost two months.

In a move, and in rhetoric that echoed those of the former apartheid government, the ANC-led government instituted dismissal procedures when the striking nurses refused to return to work. Claiming that they could not afford to pay the wage increases, the government appealed to nurses' consciences and repeatedly called on their sense of duty and their moral obligations to their patients to encourage them to suspend their strike. Gauteng Department of Health spokesperson Popo Maja said that 'workers' demands could not be met immediately, but lives had to be saved'. The director general of health further warned nurses that they could face criminal charges if patients died as a result of the strikes. President Nelson Mandela also spoke out against the strike, urging nurses to leave the profession if they were not prepared to return to work.

Nurses had legitimate grievances on all fronts and yet, in the face of government threats of mass dismissal, most of the Baragwanath nursing staff returned to work by the beginning of October. An uneasy truce was struck between the striking nurses and the government when nurses accepted that nothing would be done until the new budget in March 1996.

This strike points to the continuities in Baragwanath's history. From its inception as a civilian hospital, Baragwanath suffered from a shortage of resources. Its status as a black hospital meant that during the apartheid period it received less money per patient day than its white counterparts such as the

Johannesburg General Hospital. During the transition Baragwanath suffered a shortage of staff in the region of 30 per cent, while it was estimated that the overall shortage of staff at the Johannesburg General was about 10 per cent. This was exacerbated when HIV began to take its toll on the Baragwanath workforce in the mid-1990s. There was also vast inequity in the infrastructure and provision of equipment in apartheid times, and little was done to address these deficiencies during or immediately after the transition. The harsh reality of this situation played out everyday in the neonatal wards. If a newborn weighs less than 2.2 pounds, no extraordinary measures are taken to save the baby, even though such technology exists and is in use in better-resourced hospitals. At Baragwanath there were simply not sufficient resources to provide for all but the most viable.[19]

In other ways the period of transition brought about some significant changes. As the previous chapters have shown, almost all Baragwanath's upper-middle management and senior doctors during the apartheid era were white. This meant that the biggest reorientation for the hospital was at the senior levels of hospital administration and among the doctors. Bringing more black doctors into senior positions at the hospital was not easy. Almost five decades of inequality and oppression meant that very few black doctors had moved up though the ranks. Those with the necessary skills and training were in short supply, and demand for them was high from the public and private sectors.

The focus on nurses and on doctors does not mean that other areas of the hospital remained untransformed. However, the fact that Baragwanath already treated black patients meant that, unlike the Johannesburg General Hospital and other public and private white hospitals, Baragwanath would not experience a change in the composition of its patient body. At the same time, the major changes in the racial division of labour among nurses had occurred decades earlier, and there were already black nurses in fairly senior positions within the hospital management system. None of these groups would escape the complex process of re-evaluating and re-orientating institutional and labour relations.

It has been argued convincingly by Von Holdt and Maserumule that this process was characterised by a managerial vacuum and failure to exert disciplinary control which led in turn to a slow unravelling of workplace relations and practices and, therefore, deterioration in the quality of health care and of working life. Overwork and stress also had a very negative effect on relationships between staff and between different occupational groups; this fragmentation saw an increase in staff accusing each other of being lazy, absent without cause, drunk at work and guilty of theft and corruption.[20]

It was in these trying conditions that the hospital underwent a name change. In 1997 it became 'Chris Hani Baragwanath'. The name change had an important symbolic effect. Changing place names in South Africa has been an important marker of the reshaping of national identity. These changes seek to allow communities to reconnect with places which had names imposed on them by the colonial or apartheid regimes. Naming Baragwanath hospital after the slain anti-apartheid hero was a way of bringing the hospital firmly into the post-apartheid era – at least on the surface.

Yet the retention of 'Baragwanath' is also significant in its recognition of the mythic status of 'Bara' and in its acknowledgement that the hospital's present and future is inextricably linked to the history told in the preceding pages of this book.

The name 'Baragwanath' was part of a shared memory which had been shaped by the community within and outside its walls and had come to symbolise much more than merely the bricks and mortar of the hospital. 'Bara' was deeply intertwined with the identities of the men and women who worked there. They were 'Bara Boeties' or 'Bara Girls'. They drew on, and in some cases shaped, the mythology and ethos of the hospital as a way of claiming ownership of the situations in which they found themselves. For some this took on a political or social justice aspect; for others it was rooted in clinical practice, and yet others saw their service at Baragwanath as a calling to heal those in need. In whichever way they exercised the Baragwanath mythology and ethos, the doctors and nurses tended to refer to earlier generations of hospital staff to legitimise their claims. In this way, there was a remarkable continuity in the way that the hospital was viewed by those who worked within its wards and corridors and how they presented the hospital to the outside world. Baragwanath's doctors and nurses almost universally presented the hospital to the outside world as a positive, enriching environment (albeit one with problems) that could compete with hospitals anywhere in the world.

This view of Baragwanath and the identity and ethos its staff were said to share is, to some extent of course, rooted in nostalgia. Much of my research for the book was carried out in post-apartheid South Africa which found a number of doctors and nurses looking back to the pre-AIDS period as a kind of 'golden age' for the hospital. Yet nostalgia alone cannot explain the enduring mythology of this massive hospital.

For many doctors and nurses the legendary nature of the hospital and its unique spirit justified being there, and created a shared sense of pride in the 'Bara experience'. For doctors, the huge patient loads, severe pathology, and the ability to serve at an academic hospital but still practise outside the direct purview of the authorities did bring some real advantages to their careers, but the repeated, almost obsessive nature of these claims suggests that they could also be a coping mechanism. Faced with the hardships and trauma, they appealed to these benefits to convince themselves and others of the value of being at Baragwanath. For those whose sense of social justice or political activism led them to practise medicine, or to nursing, there could be few better places to work at than Baragwanath.

Those who worked at and identified with the hospital invested not only in their careers and their patients but also in ensuring that Baragwanath found a way to survive and thrive within the apartheid state. In this way the staff, from whichever side of the political spectrum they were on, were united in fighting a common set of adversaries. The enemy was anything that sought to impede the functioning of Baragwanath Hospital. Thus, during the apartheid era the staff at Baragwanath, as varied as they were, forged a common identity that seemed to be lost during the transition to democracy. The simmering labour tensions, leadership vacuum and overwhelming nature of work at the hospital has seemingly failed to develop a new common identity that could play a significant role in creating support structures and coping mechanisms in the current hospital.

Any account of Baragwanath would reveal the impact of apartheid on the hospital in broad brushstrokes. There is no doubt that Baragwanath was an apartheid hospital that can be seen as serving the apartheid project whereby segregated African patients were often given inferior treatment; where the funding and staffing was vastly unequal to that given to white hospitals; and where power lay in the hands of the white administration. The very nature of much of the pathology seen at the hospital was a product of the inequalities and nature of apartheid society. This is not the whole story.

Baragwanath cannot be seen as an institution in isolation. My study has shown the importance of understanding the longer-term history of the institution, for example the debates over its founding and transformation into a civilian hospital, in order to grasp the full impact these factors had on shaping its later functioning. The broader social processes occurring in South Africa at the time of the founding, and then the development of the hospital, all had an important effect on the institutional dynamics and the relationship between the hospital and its various managing authorities.

By going inside Baragwanath, my book has explored the functioning of an apartheid institution in a way that details its own internal logic, and has opened individual agency to historical scrutiny. Through an analysis of the motivations, experiences and perceptions of the institutional actors, a more nuanced picture of the daily functioning of a black apartheid hospital has emerged. Those who ran the hospital and worked in it developed their own priorities and were sometimes able to use the complex framework of health care delivery and hospital management to maximise resources. This, and the material and intellectual resources provided by the links to the medical school, created the opportunity for the development of medical specialties at Baragwanath and the possibility of advanced and highly technical care.

South Africa is in the second decade of the new millennium. The troubled phoenix of the transition has finally died and the one born into a more mature democracy has begun its life on a more hopeful note. The upgrading of infrastructure at Baragwanath is finally under way. The JD Allen Theatre Block, the Psychiatric Unit and the Paediatric Oncology unit have been renovated and expanded. In 1999 the hospital began to be computerised – and patients no longer have to protect their yellow admission files with their lives.

Endnotes

1   K Von Holdt and B Maserumule (2005) 'After Apartheid: Decay or Reconstruction? Transition in a Public Hospital'. In E Webster and K Von Holdt (eds) *Beyond the Apartheid Workplace: Studies in Transition.* Scottsville: UKZN Press, p. 4.

2   CVDH File 2, pp. 128–32.

3   CVDH, File 3, B Adair for Cheadle, Thompson and Haysom, Attorneys, Notaries and Conveyances to Dr G Marais, the minister for administration and tourism, 11 June 1992.

4   Von Holdt and Maserumule op. cit., p. 4.

5   Nehawu's proposals on Friday 12 June 1992.

6   CVDH Files 2, 17 June 1992, meeting with Mrs Langley.

7   CVDH Files 2, meeting Dr Bruwer, SANA president with Bara nurses, 25 June 1992 and Harriet Gwebu, 16 August 2003.

8   CVDH Files 3, march for workers' rights, issued by Strike Crisis Committee, nd.

9   CVDH Files 3, meeting of chief nursing service manager with self-selected 'leaders' for feedback on the two memoranda handed over by the students on 17 and 18 July 1992.

10   CVDH Files 2, Cheadle, Thompson and Haysom, Attorneys, Notaries and Conveyancers to Dr G Marais, minister for Administration and Tourism, 11 June 1992.

11   CVDH File 3, National Education Health and Allied Workers Union.

12   CVDH Files 3, Re: Burnet House, statement by LM Makgotloe, 16 August 1991.

13   CVDH File 3, Intimidation and Violence, Bara Health Workers Crisis Committee.

14   Von Holdt and Maserumule op. cit.

15   CVDH Files, File 2, 'Recognition and Procedural Agreement between the Transvaal Provincial Administration (TPA) and National Education, Health and Allied Workers Union (Nehawu)', 1 February 1993, p. 4.

16   Nehawu's proposals on Friday 12 June 1992.

17   'Conflicting Views of the Hospital Dispute', *Saturday Star*, 20 June 1992.

18   Von Holdt and Maserumule op. cit., p. 14.

19   Bell op. cit., p. 1.

20   Von Holdt and Maserumule op. cit., p. 5.

Bibliography

Archival sources

Adler Museum of Medicine (Adler Museum), Wits Faculty of Health Sciences, Johannesburg.

Baragwanath Hospital Board Minutes (BHBM), in the possession of the Baragwanath Hospital secretary, Chris Hani Baragwanath Hospital, Soweto.

Baragwanath Hospital Department of Medicine Files and Archives (DMF), in the possession of the head of the Department of Medicine, Chris Hani Baragwanath Hospital, Soweto.

Baragwanath Hospital Public Relations Archives (Bara PR Archives), in the possession of the Public Relations Department, Chris Hani Baragwanath Hospital, Soweto.

Central Archive Depot, Pretoria National Archive (SAB).

Dubb Papers, in the possession of Professor Asher Dubb, Johannesburg.

Kaplan Papers, in the possession of Yehuda Kaplan, Rotherham, England.

University of the Witwatersrand, Central Archives and Registry (Wits Archives), Johannesburg.

University of the Witwatersrand, Faculty of Health Science Registry (WHSR), Johannesburg.

University of the Witwatersrand, Faculty of Health Sciences Library (WHSL), Johannesburg.

University of the Witwatersrand, Historical Papers Collection (HPW), William Cullen Library, Johannesburg.

Van den Heever Papers (VdH Papers), in the possession of Chris van den Heever, Johannesburg.

Bibliography

A Brief History of Health Workers' Struggles in South Africa. *Critical Health* 15, May 1986.

An Historical Overview of Nursing Struggles in South Africa. *Critical Health* 24, October 1998.

Abel R (1995) *Politics by Other Means: Law in the Struggle Against Apartheid.* New York: Routledge.

Altmann A (1948) 'Malignant Malnutrition, Kwashiorkor'. *Clinical Proceedings* 7.

Altmann A (1953) 'Kwashiorkor, Malignant Malnutrition – Infantile Pellagra'. *South African Journal of Clinical Science* 4:2, June.

Altmann A and CG Anderson (1951) 'Electrophoretic Serum Protein Pattern in Malignant Malnutrition'. *Lancet* 1:4, January.

Anderson N and S Marks (1988) 'Apartheid and Health in the 1980s'. *Social Science and Medicine* 27.

Anderson N and S Marks (1989) 'The State, Class and the Allocation of Health Resources in Southern Africa'. *Social Science and Medicine* 28.

Annual Report of the Department of Public Health, Year Ending 30 June 1928, UG 47-

Annual Report of the Department of Public Health, Year Ending 30 June 1974, RP 34-

Arnold D (ed.) (1996) *Warm Climates and Western Medicine; the Emergence of Tropical Medicine, 1500–1900.* Amsterdam: Rodopi.

'Badges on the Cover'. *South African Nurses Journal* 61:4, April 1974.

Baldwin-Ragaven L, J de Gruchy and L London (1999) *An Ambulance of the Wrong Colour: Health Professionals, Human Rights and Ethics in South Africa.* Cape Town: UCT Press.

'Baragwanath Hospital Strike 1985: Divided Interests and Joint Action'. *Critical Health* May 1986.

Baragwanath Hospital Yearbook 1992/3.

'Baragwanath – Place of Healing'. *South African Panorama* January 1967.

'Baragwanath: The People's Hospital'. *Southern Africa Today* July 1986.

Barold S (1996) 'Leo Schamroth (1924–1988): His Life and Work'. *Journal of Medical Biographies* 4:3, August.

Beinart W (2001) *Twentieth-Century South Africa.* Oxford: Oxford University Press.

Bell CW (1998) 'World's Largest Hospital Juggles Limited Resources to Deliver Adequate Care'. *Modern Healthcare* 28, May.

Benatar SR (1991) 'Medicine and Health Care in South Africa – Five Years Later'. *New England Journal of Medicine* 325:1, July.

Benatar SR and RE Kirsch (1987) 'Baragwanath – a Hospital in Despair'. *South African Medical Journal* 72, September.

Beukes PJ (2004) 'The Birth and First 10 Years of Primary Health Care in Soweto' (unpublished paper).

Beukes PJ (2005) 'The Day Hector Peterson Died, by the Soweto from Namaqualand' (unpublished manuscript, in Beukes's possession).

Blumsohn D (1994) 'The Pathology of Poverty'. In K Huddle and A Dubb (eds) *Baragwanath Hospital: 50 Years, A Medical Miscellany*. Johannesburg: Department of Medicine, Baragwanath Hospital.

Bonner P and L Segal (1998) *Soweto: A History*. Cape Town: Maskew Miller Longman.

Botha E (1988) 'A Bara Person'. *Publico* 8:2, April.

Bothwell TM (1993) 'Some Aspects of Research at Baragwanath Hospital in its Early Years'. *Adler Museum Bulletin* 19:2, July.

Brandel-Syrier M (1971) *Reeftown Elite: A Study of Social Mobility in a Modern African Community on the Reef*. London: Routledge & Kegan Paul.

Bremner CG (1971) 'The Changing Pattern of Disease seen at Baragwanath Hospital'. *South African Journal of Surgery* 9:3, July–September.

Bremner CG (1998) 'Modern Surgery in Africa: The Baragwanath Experience: A Book Review'. *South African Journal of Science* 84:11, November.

Brink E, G Malungane, D Ntshangase, B Mnguni and S Lebelo (2001) *Soweto 16 June 1976: It All Started with a Dog*. Cape Town: Kwela.

Browde J, E Jassat and P Mokhobo (1998) Internal Reconciliation Commission: Faculty of Health Sciences, University of the Witwatersrand, Summary Report.

Burke T (1996) *Lifebuoy Men, Lux Women: Commodification, Consumption and Cleanliness in Modern Zimbabwe*. London: Duke University Press.

Burrows EH (1958) *A History of Medicine in South Africa up to the End of the Nineteenth Century*. Cape Town: Balkema.

Butchart A (1997) 'The "Bantu Clinic": A Genealogy of the African Patient as Object and Effect of South African Clinical Medicine, 1930–1990'. *Culture, Medicine and Psychiatry* 21.

Butchart A (1998) *The Anatomy of Power: European Constructions of the African Body*. London: Zed.

Cajee I (2005) *Timol – Quest for Justice: Ahmed Timol's Life and Martyrdom*. Johannesburg: STE.

Caldwell RA (1957) 'In Memoriam'. *South African Medical Journal* 31.

Carmichael L (2004) *Friendship: Interpreting Christian Love*. London: T & T Clark International.

Carr, WJP (1990) *Soweto: Its Creation, Life and Decline*. Johannesburg: South African Institute of Race Relations.

Carther T (1985) 'Baragwanath Hospital'. *The Medical Journal of Australia* 142, April.

Charlewood GP (1948) 'Cardiac Arrest: Modified Technique of Cardiac Massage'. *British Medical Journal* 2, December.

Charlewood GP (1949) 'False Vagina Formed by Coitus'. *The Journal of Obstetrics and Gynaecology of the British Empire* 56:2.

Charlewood GP (1956) *Bantu Gynaecology*. Johannesburg: Photo Pub. Co. of SA.

Charlewood GP, S Shippel and H Renton (1949) 'Schistosomiasis in Gynaecology'. *The Journal of Obstetrics and Gynaecology of the British Empire* 56:3.

Cheater AP (1974) 'A Marginal Elite? African Registered Nurses in Durban, South Africa'. *African Studies* 33.

City of Johannesburg *Annual Report of the Medical Officer of Health* 1940–1955.

City of Johannesburg *Mayor's Minutes* 1930–1940.

Committee to Inquire into the Training of Natives in Medicine and Public Health, Loram Committee, UG 35–28 Pretoria.

'Conditions at Baragwanath Hospital'. *South African Medical Journal* 72, September 1987.

Connor, JTH (1990) 'Review Essay: Hospital History in Canada and the United States'. *Canadian Bulletin of Medical History* 7:93–104.

Cooper M (1958) 'New Pattern of Protest'. *Contact: The SA News Review* 1:5, April.

Cousins B (1990) 'Heroes in White'. *Adler Museum Bulletin* 16:2, July.

Dart R (1937) 'Racial Origins'. In Schapera I (ed.) *The Bantu Speaking Tribes of South Africa*. London: George Routledge & Sons.

De Beer C (1986) *The South African Disease: Apartheid Health and Health Services*. London: Africa World Press.

De Beer C (1988) *How Many Beds Does Baragwanath Hospital Need?* Johannesburg: Centre For the Study of Health Policy, Department of Community Health, University of the Witwatersrand.

De Beer J (1976) 'A Forward View of Health Services in South Africa', *South African Medical Journal* 50:11, March.

Deacon H, P Howard and E van Heyningen (eds) (2004), *The Cape Doctor in the Nineteenth Century: A Social History*. Amsterdam: Rodopi.

Dellatola L (1977) 'Soweto's Healers'. *Panorama,* February.

Digby A (1999) *The Evolution of British General Practice 1850–1940*. Oxford: Oxford University Press.

DigbyA (2005) 'Early Black Doctors in South Africa'. *Journal of African History* 46:3.

Digby A and H Sweet (2002) 'Nurses as Cultural Brokers in Twentieth-Century South Africa'. In Ernst W (ed.) *Plural Medicine, Tradition and Modernity, 1800–2000*. London: Routledge.

Digby A, H Phillip, H Deacon and K Tomson (2008) *At the Heart of Healing in Cape Town: Groote Schuur Hospital, 1938–2008*. Johannesburg: Jacana.

Dreger AD (1988) 'The Limits of Individuality: Ritual and Sacrifice in the Lives and Medical Treatment of Conjoined Twins'. *Studies in the History and Philosophy of Biology and Biomedical Science* 29.

Drummond G, P Scott, D Mackay and R Lipschitz (1991) 'Separation of the Baragwanath Craniopagus Twins'. *British Journal of Plastic Surgery* 44:1, January.

Dubb A (1988) 'Baragwanath Hospital 1948–1972: The Department of Medicine: The First 25 Years'. *Adler Museum Bulletin* 24:1/2, July.

Dubow S (1995) *Scientific Racism in Modern South Africa*. Cambridge: Cambridge University Press.

Dubow S (2006) *A Commonwealth of Knowledge: Science, Sensibility, and White South Africa, 1820–2000*. Oxford: Oxford University Press.

Du Toit D (1981) *Capital and Labour in South Africa: Class Struggle in the 1970s*. London: Kegan Paul International.

Du Preez Bezdrob AM (2001) *Winnie Mandela: A Life*. Cape Town: New Holland.

Dyason D (1988) 'The Medical Profession in Colonial Victoria'. In MacLeod R and M Lewis (eds) *Disease, Medicine and Empire: Perspectives on Western Medicine and the Experience of European Expansion*. London: Routledge.

Edelstein W (1971) 'The Management of Transverse Lie in Labour'. *South African Journal of Obstetrics and Gynecology* 4, May.

Eisenstein (1977) 'The Morphology and Pathological Anatomy of Lumber Spine in South African Negro and Caucasoid with Specific Reference to Spinal Stenosis'. *Journal of Bone Joint Surgery* 59:2, May.

Fassin D (2007) *When Bodies Remember: Experiences and Politics of AIDS in South Africa*. Berkeley: University of California Press.

Fatti L and JC Gilroy (1949) 'Thoracoscopy as an Aid to Diagnosis in Congenital Heart Disease'. *The British Heart Journal* 11:3.

Feasby WR (1953) *Official History of the Canadian Medical Services, 1939–1945: Organization and Campaigns*. Ottawa: Cloutier.

Forsyth G (1973) *Doctors and State Medicine: A Study of the British Health Service*. London: Forsyth.

Foucault M (1973) *The Birth of the Clinic*. London: Pantheon.

Frack I (1958a) 'Guest Editorial: Baragwanath Hospital, Decennial Anniversary'. *Medical Proceedings* 4:10, May.

Frack I (1958b) 'In Memoriam: John Donald Allen OBE 1900–1957'. *Medical Proceedings* 4:10, May.

Frack I (1970) *Every Man Must Play a Part: The Story of a South African Doctor*. Cape Town: Purnell.

Franklin J and C Hatzitheofilou (1987) 'Arteriovenous Fistulas and False Aneurysms Occurring after Trauma'. *South African Journal of Surgery* 25:3, September.

French K (1983) 'James Mpanza and the Sofasonke Party in the Development of Local Politics in Soweto'. University of the Witwatersrand, MA thesis.

Freund W (2007) 'South Africa as Developmental State'. *Africanus: Journal of Development Studies* 37:2.

Gear JH (1965) 'The Johannesburg Hospital: A Historical Outline of the First Fifty Years'. *South African Medical Journal* 39.

Girard CSM (1983) 'Canadian Nurses in the South African Military Nursing Service: Some Reminiscences Forty Years Later'. *Military History Journal* 6:1, June.

Giraud RMA, I Luke and A Schmaman (1969) 'Crohn's Disease in the Transvaal Bantu: A Report of 5 Cases'. *South African Medical Journal* 43:21, May.

Goodman T and M Price (1999) 'Using an Internal Reconciliation Commission to Facilitate Organisational Change in Post-Apartheid South Africa – The Case of Wits Health Science Faculty' (unpublished paper).

Granshaw L (1997) 'The Hospital'. In Bynum WF and R Porter (1997) *Companion Encyclopaedia of the History of Medicine*. London: Routledge.

Granshaw L and R Porter (1989) *The Hospital in History*. London: Routledge.

Grusin H (1955) 'Potassium Dichromate as a Witchdoctor's Remedy: Five Cases of Poisoning'. *South African Medical Journal* 29:6, February.

Grusin H and PS Kincaid-Smith (1954) 'Scurvy in Adult Africans: A Clinical, Hematological, and Pathological Study'. *American Journal of Clinical Nutrition* 2:5, September–October.

Harris SE (1951) 'The British Health Experiment: The First Two Years of the National Health Service'. *The American Economic Review* 41:2, May.

Harrison N (1985) *Winnie Mandela: Mother of a Nation*. London: Gollancz.

Hebestreit L (1969) 'Nursing Service and Education at Baragwanath Hospital'. *South African Medical Journal* 43:21, May.

Hellmann E (1948) *Rooiyard: A Sociological Study of an Urban Slumyard*. Oxford: Oxford University Press.

Hellmann E (1971) *Soweto: Johannesburg's African City*. Johannesburg: South African Institute of Race Relations.

Higginson J (1951) 'Malignant Neoplastic Disease in the South African Bantu'. *Cancer* 4:6, November.

Higginson J (1953) 'Study of Malignant Neoplastic Disease in Primitive Communities with Special Reference to South Africa'. *South African Medical Journal* 27:17, April.

Higginson J (1956) 'Primary Carcinoma of the Liver in Africa'. *British Journal of Cancer* 10:4, December.

Hine DC (1989) *Black Women in White: Racial Conflict and Cooperation in the Nursing Profession, 1890–1950*. Bloomington: Indiana University Press.

Hirson B (1979) *Year of Ash, Year of Fire. The Soweto Revolt: Roots of a Revolution?* London: Zed.

Hirsowits L (1948) 'Typhoid Fever in the Bantu' (University of the Witwatersrand MD thesis).

Hospital and Nursing Yearbook of Southern Africa. Johannesburg, 1950–1990.

Huddle K and A Dubb (eds) (1994) *Baragwanath Hospital, 50 Years: A Medical Miscellany*. Johannesburg: Department of Medicine, Baragwanath Hospital.

Hunt JA (2002) *White Witchdoctor: A Surgeon's Life in Apartheid South Africa.* Dallas: Durban House.

Hyslop J (1999) *The Classroom Struggle: Policy and Resistance in South Africa 1940–1990.* Scottsville: University of Natal Press.

Issacson C (1977) 'Changing Patterns of Heart Disease in South African Blacks'. *South African Medical Journal* 52:20, November.

Jarrett-Kerr M (1961) *African Pulse: Scenes from an African Hospital Window.* London: Morehouse-Barlow.

Jeeves A (2001) 'Public Health in the Era of South Africa's Syphilis Epidemic of the 1930s and 1940s'. *South African Historical Journal* 45.

Jochelson K (2001) *The Colour of Disease: Syphilis and Racism in South Africa, 1880–1950.* Basingstoke: Palgrave.

Johannesburg City Council, *Johannesburg City Council Minutes,* 1920–1950.

Johnson J and P Magubane (1981) *Soweto Speaks.* Johannesburg: AD Donker.

Joseph H (1986) *Side by Side: The Autobiography of Helen Joseph.* London: Morrow.

Keeley KJ (1958) 'Alimentary Disease in the Bantu', *Medical Proceedings,* 4:10, May.

Kelly J (1990) *Finding a Cure: The Politics of Health in South Africa.* Johannesburg: South African Institute of Race Relations.

Kenny WHF (1969) 'Baragwanath Hospital's Twenty-First Birthday'. *South African Medical Journal* 43:21, May.

Kentron TO (1958) 'Anti-Apartheid Nursing Body to Confer: Protest Against Act Growing'. *Contact: The SA News Review,* June.

Kleinot S (1958) 'The Work of the Surgical Division'. *Medical Proceedings* 4:10, May: 286–92.

Kuper H (1965) 'Nurses'. In Kuper L *An African Bourgeoisie: Race, Class, and Politics in South Africa.* New Haven: Yale University Press.

Laden S (2003) 'Who's Afraid of the Black Bourgeoisie? Consumer Magazines for Black South Africans as an Apparatus of Change'. *Journal of Consumer Culture* 3: 191–216.

Laidler PW and M Gelfand (1971) *South Africa: Its Medical History, 1652–1898.* Cape Town: Struik.

Lawson HH (1988) Preface, in D Pantanowitz (ed.) *Modern Surgery in Africa: The Baragwanath Experience.* Johannesburg: Southern.

Lawson HH (1994) 'The Department of Surgery, Baragwanath Hospital – the Early Days', *South African Journal of Surgery* 32:1, March.

Lee NC (1988) 'Bara: an Editorial Dilemma'. *South African Medical Journal* 73:8, April.

Levin S (1989) 'Siamese Twins: Double Trouble'. *Nursing RSA* 4:7, July.

Lewis P (1969) *'City Within a City': The Creation of Soweto*. Johannesburg: Wits University Press.

Lipschitz R (1967) 'Associated Injuries and Complications of Stab Wounds of the Spinal Cord'. *Paraplegia* 5:2, August.

Lipschitz R and J Block (1962) 'Stab Wounds of the Spinal Cord'. *Lancet* 2, July.

Lodge T and W Nasson (1992) *All Here and Now: Black Politics in South Africa in the 1980s*. London: Foreign Policy Association.

Longmore L (1959) *The Dispossessed: A Study of the Sex-life of Bantu Women in Urban Areas in and around Johannesburg*. London: Cape.

Loughlin K (2005) 'Spectacle and Secrecy: Press Coverage of Conjoined Twins in 1950s Britain'. *Medical History* 49.

Mager AK (1999) *Gender and the Making of a South African Bantustan: A Social History of the Ciskei, 1945–1959*. Johannesburg: Heinemann.

Makhetha P (1989) 'The Matibela Siamese Twins'. *Nursing RSA* 4:7, July.

Malan M (1988) *In Quest of Health: The South African Institute for Medical Research, 1912–1973*. Johannesburg: Lowry Publishers.

Marks S (1994) *Divided Sisterhood: Race, Class and Gender in the South African Nursing Profession*. London: St. Martin's Press.

Marks S (1997a) 'South Africa's Early Experiment in Social Medicine, Its Pioneers and Politics'. *American Journal of Public Health* 87.

Marks S (1997b) 'The Legacy of the History of Nursing for Post-apartheid South Africa. In Rafferty AM, J Robinson and R Elkan (eds) *Nursing History and the Politics of Welfare* (New York: Routledge).

Marks S (1997c) 'What is Colonial about Colonial Medicine? And What Has Happened to Imperial Health?' *Social History of Medicine* 10.

Marks S and N Andersson (1984) 'Epidemics and Social Control in Twentieth Century South Africa'. *The Society for the Social History of Medicine Bulletin* 34.

Marks S and N Andersson (1987) 'Issues in the Political Economy of Health in Southern Africa'. *Journal of Southern African Studies* 13.

Martin HJ and N Orpen (1979) *South Africa at War, Military and Industrial Organization and Operations in Connection with the Conduct of the War, 1939–1945*. Cape Town: Purnell.

Mashaba TG (1995) *Rising to the Challenge of Change: A History of Black Nursing in South Africa*. Cape Town: Juta.

Maud JP (1938) *City Government: The Johannesburg Experiment*. Oxford: Clarendon Press.

McLean GR and T Jenkins (2003) 'The Steve Biko Affair: A Case Study in Medical Ethics'. *Developing World Bioethics*, 3:1, May.

Medical Graduates Association, University of the Witwatersrand 'Conditions at Baragwanath'. *South African Medical Journal* 73, April 1988.

Meerkotter DV and J Craig (1988) 'Spinal Stenosis at Baragwanath Hospital, Johannesburg'. *South African Journal of Surgery*, 26:1, March.

Miller P and R Lipschitz (1987) 'Transclival Penetrating Injury'. *Neurosurgery* 21:1, July.

Moran B, A Webb-Johnson and E Holland (1946) 'Correspondence: Demobilised Specialists'. *British Medical Journal* 2, July.

Morris P (1981) 'Soweto: A Brief History'. *The Black Sash* 24:2, August.

Motsapi I (1987) 'These Babies are a Gift from God, says Mother'. *Bona* June.

Murray B (1997) *Wits, The Open Years: A History of the University of the Witwatersrand*, Johannesburg, 1939–1959. Johannesburg: Wits University Press.

Murray BK (1990) 'Wits as an "Open" University 1939–1959: Black Admission to the University of the Witwatersrand'. *Journal of Southern African Studies* 16, December.

Nicholson GWL (1975) *Canada's Nursing Sisters*. Toronto: S Stevens.

Noble V (2005) 'Doctors Divided: Gender, Race and Class Anomalies in the Production of Black Medical Doctors in Apartheid South Africa, 1948–1994'. University of Michigan PhD thesis.

'Obituary: In Memoriam – Jane McLarty (1893–1989)'. *Nursing RSA* 4:3, March 1989.

'Obituary: Sister Dora Nginza'. *South African Nursing Journal* 3:8, August 1966.

Olivier LR and JR Kriel (1978) 'A Job Well Done – A Short History of Dr James Moroka'. *South African Medical Journal* 54:8, August.

'Other Strikes at Other Hospitals'. *Critical Health* 15, May 1986.

Packard R (1987) 'Tuberculosis and the Development of Industrial Health Policies'. *Journal of Southern African Studies* 13.

Packard R (1990) *White Plague, Black Labour: Tuberculosis and the Political Economy of Health and Disease in South Africa*. Scottsville: University of Natal Press.

Pantanowitz D (ed.) (1988) *Modern Surgery in Africa: The Baragwanath Experience*. Johannesburg: Southern.

Pantanowitz D (1994) *Alternative Medicine: A Doctor's Perspective*. Cape Town: Southern.

Parekh D and HH Lawson (1987) 'Gallstone Disease among Black South Africans: A Review of the Baragwanath Hospital Experience'. *South African Medical Journal* 72:1, July.

Pauw BA (1963) *The Second Generation: A Study of the Family among Urbanised Bantu in East London*. London: Oxford University Press.

Petersen EW (1958) 'African Nurse Training – Ten Years of Progress'. *Medical Proceedings* 4:10, May.

Phillips H (1990) *Black October: The Influence of the Spanish Influenza Epidemic of 1918 on South Africa*. Pretoria: Government Printer.

Phillips R (1938) *The Bantu in the City: A Study of Cultural Adjustment on the Witwatersrand*. Alice: Lovedale Press.

Pickstone PV (1985) *Medicine and Industrial Society: A History of Hospital Development in Manchester and its Region, 1752–1946*. Manchester: Manchester University Press.

Porter R (1985) 'The Patient's View: Doing Medical History from Below'. *Theory and Society*, 14.

Porter R and D Porter (1989) *Patient's Progress: Doctors and Doctoring in Eighteenth-Century England*. Cambridge: Cambridge University Press.

Posel D (1997) *The Making of Apartheid, 1948–1961: Conflict and Compromise*. Oxford: Clarendon Press.

Rabinowitz B and D Demetriades (1988) 'Resuscitation'. In Pantanowitz (ed.) *Modern Surgery in Africa: The Baragwanath Experience*. Johannesburg: Southern.

Report of the Hospital Survey Committee. Thornton Committee, UG 25-1927 (Pretoria, 1927).

Report of the Inter-Departmental Committee on the Social Health and Economic Conditions of Urban Natives. Smit Committee, GP 57272-1942-3 (Pretoria, 1942).

Report of the National Health Services Commission on the Provision of an Organised National Health Services for All Sectors of the People of the

Union of South Africa. Gluckman Commission, UG 30-44 (Pretoria, 1944).

Resha M (1991) *'Mangoana O Tsoara Thipa ka Bohaleng': My Life in the Struggle.* Johannesburg: COSAW.

Rispel L and M Motsei (1998) 'Nurses and Their Work – A Survey of Opinions'. *Critical Health* 24, October.

Risse GB (1999) *Mending Bodies, Saving Souls: A History of Hospitals.* Oxford: Oxford University Press.

Rivett G (1986) *Development of the London Hospital System, 1823–1982.* London: Oxford University Press.

Rosenberg C (1987) *The Care of Strangers: The Rise of America's Hospital System.* New York: Basic Books.

Rosenberg CE (1978) 'Inward Vision and Outward Glance: The Shaping of the American Hospital, 1880–1914'. *Bulletin of the History of Medicine* 53.

Saadia R (1999) 'Organisation of Hospital Responses for the Trauma Epidemic'. *British Medical Bulletin* 55:4.

Saffer D and G Modi (1994) 'Neurology'. In Dubb A and K Huddle (eds) *Baragwanath Hospital: 50 Years, A Medical Miscellany.* Johannesburg: Department of Medicine, Baragwanath Hospital.

Sakalo W (1979) 'Letter from … Soweto, Baragwanath Hospital, 1978'. *British Medical Journal* 1, March.

Schamroth L (1971) *The Disorders of Cardiac Rhythm.* Oxford: Blackwell Scientific Publications.

Schamroth L (1984) *Electrocardiology of Coronary Artery Disease.* Oxford: Blackwell Scientific Publications.

Schamroth L (1989) *Twelve Lead Electrocardiography.* Oxford: Blackwell Scientific Publications.

Schwartz MB, L Schamroth and HC Seftel (1958) 'The Pattern of Heart Disease in the Urbanised (Johannesburg) African'. *Medical Proceedings* 4:10, May.

Searle C (1965) *The History of the Development of Nursing in South Africa.* Cape Town: Struik.

Seedat A (1984) *Crippling a Nation: Health in Apartheid South Africa.* London: International Defence and Aid Fund for Southern Africa.

Segal I (1988) 'The Trauma of the Urban Experience'. *Journal of the Royal College of Physicians London* 22:1, January.

Segal I and JA Hunt (1975) 'The Irritable Bowel Syndrome in the Urban South African Negro'. *South African Medical Journal* 49:40, September.

Segal I and LO Tim (1979) 'The Witchdoctor and the Bowel'. *South African Medical Journal* 56:8, August.

Segal I, LO Tim, A Solomon and A Giraud (1978) 'Diverticular Disease in Urban Blacks'. *South African Medical Journal* 53:23, June: 922.

Segal I, ARP Walker and D Parekh (1994) 'Gastroenterology. In Huddle K and A Dubb (eds) *Baragwanath Hospital, 50 Years: A Medical Miscellany.* Johannesburg: Department of Medicine, Baragwanath Hospital.

Senokoanyane N (1995) *Their Light, Love and Life: A Black Nurse's Story*. Cape Town: Kwela.

Shapiro KA (1987) 'Doctors or Medical Aids: The Debate over the Training of Black Medical Personnel for the Rural Black Population in South Africa in the 1920s and 1930s'. *Journal of Southern African Studies* 13.

Shimoni G (2003) *Community and Conscience, Jews in Apartheid South Africa*. London: University Press of New England.

Sigerist HE (1936) 'An Outline of the Development of the Hospital'. *Bulletin of the History of Medicine* 4.

Simpson AW (1958) 'Nursing Services at the Baragwanath Hospital'. *Medical Proceedings* 4:10, May.

Skapinker W (1949) 'Intestinal Obstruction due to Ascaris'. *British Journal of Surgery* 37:145.

Smith J (1989) 'Baragwanath: the Squalor of Segregation'. *British Medical Journal* 298, March.

South African Nursing Journal, 1960–1978.

Southall R (2006) 'Can South Africa be a Developmental State?' In Buhlungu S et al. (eds) *State of the Nation: South Africa 2005–2006*. Cape Town: HSRC Press.

Stadler AW (1979) 'Birds in the Cornfields: African Squatter Movements in Johannesburg, 1944–1947'. *Journal of Southern African Studies* 6.

Stein H and EU Rosen (1980) 'Changing Trends in Child Health in Soweto: The Baragwanath Hospital Picture'. *South African Medical Journal* 58:26, December.

Stevens R (1989) *In Sickness and in Wealth: American Hospitals in the Twentieth Century*. New York: Basic Books.

Stoler AL (2002) *Carnal Knowledge and Imperial Power: Race and the Intimate in Colonial Rule*. Berkeley: University of California Press.

Stratford DO (1969) 'Canadian Associations with the South African Military Nursing Service'. *South African Nursing Journal* 36:3, March.

Supreme Court of South Africa (Appellate Division): [zRPz]Administrator, Transvaal, and Others v. Traub and Others 1989 (4) SA 731 (A).

Swanson MW (1977) 'The Sanitation Syndrome: Bubonic Plague and Urban Native Policy in the Cape Colony'. *Journal of African History* 18.

Sweet H (2004) '"Wanted: 16 Nurses of the Better Educated Type": Provision of Nurses to South Africa in the Late Nineteenth and Early Twentieth Centuries'. *Nursing Inquiry* 11.

Sweet H and A Digby (2005) 'Race, Identity and the Nursing Profession in South Africa, c. 1850–1958'. In Mortimer B and S McCann (eds) *New Directions in the History of Nursing in International Perspective*. London: Routledge.

Swilling M and M Phillips (1989) 'State Power in the 1980s: From "Total Strategy" to Counter-Revolutionary Warfare'. In Cock J and L Nathan (eds) *War and Society: the Militarisation of South Africa*. Cape Town: Thorold.

Taylor J (1997) *The Architect and the Pavilion Hospital: Dialogue and Design Creativity in England 1859–1914*. London: Leicester University Press.

Transvaal Provincial Administration *Report of the Director of Hospital Services* (12th report), 1969–1970.

Transvaal Provincial Administration *Transvaal Provincial Administration, 1910–1986*.

'Troops Must Get Out'. *SASPU National* 12 December 1985.

Truth and Reconciliation Commission of South Africa: Final Report, Cape Town, 1998.

Turshen M (1984) *The Political Ecology of Disease in Tanzania*. New Brunswick: Rutgers University Press.

Union of South Africa Census 1946, Vol. 1, UG 51-1949 (Pretoria, 1949).

Uys L (1987) 'Racism and the South African Nurse'. *Nursing RSA*, 2:11/12, November–December.

Van Dellen JR and R Lipschitz (1978) 'Stab Wounds of the Skull'. *Surgical Neurology* 10:2, August.

Van den Heever C (1987) 'New Hope for Siamese Twins'. *Transhosp Nuus/ News* 4:1, December.

Van den Heever C (1991) 'Baragwanath, Africa's Largest Hospital'. *Africa Business and Chamber of Commerce Review* (Medical Supplement) 27:17, January.

Van den Heever C (1993) 'Baragwanath Hospital – the Beginning'. *Adler Museum Bulletin* 19:1, March.

Van den Heever C (1994) 'A History of Baragwanath Hospital'. In Huddle K and A Dubb (eds) *Baragwanath Hospital: 50 Years, A Medical Miscellany*. Johannesburg: Department of Medicine, Baragwanath Hospital.

Van Dijck J (2002) 'Medical Documentary: Conjoined Twins as a Medical Spectacle'. *Media, Culture and Society* 24.

Van Rensburg HCJ, Fourie A and E Pretorius (1992) *Health Care in South Africa: Structure and Dynamics*. Pretoria: Academica.

Van Wyk H (1987) 'Conditions at Baragwanath'. *South African Medical Journal* 72, November.

Vaughan M (1991) *Curing Their Ills: Colonial Power and African Illness*. Palo Alto: Stanford University Press.

Von Holdt K and B Maserumule (2005) 'After Apartheid: Decay or Reconstruction? Transition in a Public Hospital'. In Webster E and C von Holdt (eds) *Beyond the Apartheid Workplace: Studies in Transition*. Scottsville: UKZN Press.

Wagstaff LA (1978) 'The Changing Role of Doctors in the Soweto Clinics' Health Care Teams'. *South African Medical Journal* 53:20, May.

Wagstaff LA and PJ Beukes (1977) 'The Paediatric Primary Health Care Nurse Project in Soweto'. *South African Medical Journal* 52:27, December.

Walker AR and I Segal (1979) 'Epidemiology of Noninfective Intestinal Diseases in Various Ethnic Groups in South Africa'. *Israel Journal of Medical Sciences* 15:4, April.

Walker AR and I Segal (1979) 'Is Appendicitis Increasing in South African Blacks?' *South African Medical Journal* 56:13, September.

Webster C (1988) *The Health Services since the War*. London: HMSO.

Webster C (1990) *The National Health Service: A Political History*. Oxford: Oxford University Press.

Williams AW (1946) 'Correspondence: Demobilised Specialists'. *British Medical Journal* 2, December.

Wilson F (1972) *Labour in the South African Gold Mines 1911–1969*. Cambridge: Cambridge University Press.

Wilson TD (1984) 'Health Services within Soweto', Second Carnegie Inquiry into Poverty and Development in Southern Africa, Paper No. 170, 13–19 April.

Wilson VH (1958) 'Ten Years' Medical Experience at Baragwanath Non-European Hospital'. *Medical Proceedings* 4:10, May.

Index

Please note: Page numbers in italics refer to tables and figures.

neonatal wards   207
neurosurgery   94, 176
New Canada Hospital   188
New China News Agency   173
Ngcwabe, Zolela   184
Nginza, Dora   125
Nightingale, Florence   37
Nokuphila hospital (Seventh Day
        Adventists) 35
Non-European Affairs Department
        (NEAD)   62, 63
    armed police and road
        blocks   147–8
Non-European Hospital,
        Johannesburg   29, 30, 34,
        42, 76, 125
non-striking workers   203–4
Noordgesig township   32
Ntoko, Edith   125
nurses   19, 21, 178
    black   39–40, 59, 74–81
    Canadian   37–8
    coloured   79
    funded education   22
    Indian   79
    to patients ratio   178
    as role models   133–4
    students and juniors, militant
        action   203
    training at mission institutes   75
    see also strikes
nursing
    changes in policy   205–6
    own identities   132–3
    as part of 'civilising project' 124
    professional prestige   131

status in community   125
struggle for control of at
        Baragwanath   74–81
style, image and class   135
symbol of class and status   133
uplifting families   124
see also black women and nursing
        experience
Nursing Act (1944)   146
Nursing Act (1978)   151
Nursing Amendment Act
        (1957)   102, 146, 148
Nursing Association   151
nutrition, poor   88
nutritional deficiencies in
        children   162
Nzima, Sam   6

obstetrical nursing posts   120
operating theatre technique   141
orientation programmes   138
Orlando   30, 31, 35
    Advisory Board   59
orthopaedic nursing courses   141
Orthopaedic Spinal Unit,
        Baragwanath   91
Ou-Tim, Leonard   90
overcrowding   23, 27, 42, 64, 74,
        161, 165, 178, 180, 186,
        188–9
    and advanced medical care   162
    patient numbers   142–3
    and underresourced wards   179
'Overcrowding at Baragwanath'
        cartoon   161, 161
overwork   207–8

public sector
  costs of medical care 91
  health workers 202
Public Service Act (1984) 184
Public Works Department (PWD)
pulmonary diseases 46
PWD, see Public Works Department

race 75, 100–1
  and geographical area 56–7
racial difference
  in disease profiles 91
  and epidemiology 48
racial mixing
  and cooperation 18
  social 99
racial segregation in nursing
      legislation 146
racial tensions, heightened 151
Raikes, Humphrey 69
Ramaboa, Jane 59
Ramogole, Virginia 129–30, 135,
      137, 139
RDP, see Reconstruction and
      Development Programme
Reconstruction and Development
      Programme (RDP) 205
Red Cross 36, 38
Rees, Helen 103
Reitz Commission 15
religion 107–8
religious calling to enter nursing 123
religious motivations 113
religious sisterhoods 37
replacement workers and army
      medics 202
research 46–9, 73–4, 89

clinical 88
  and teaching 188
Resha, Maggie 79, 125, 133
resources
  allocation and priorities 167
  lack of 92
  shortages 206–7
Richter, Anna Marie 110
rickets, deficiency disease 88
Risse, Guenter
      Mending Bodies, Saving Souls 11
Roscher, Iris 154
Russell, Moira 73, 91, 150–1

Saadia, Roger 92
SADF, see South African Defence
      Force
Sadnu, see South African Democratic
      Nurses Union
SAIMR, see South African Institute of
      Medical Research
salaries
  of black mineworkers 128
  of black nurses 127–8
  of white, coloured, Indian
      counterparts 128
Saloojee, Haroon 64, 72, 95, 98,
      100, 105–6, 166, 176–7
SAMDC, see South African Medical
      and Dental Council
SANA, see South African Nursing
      Association
SANC, see South African Nursing
      Council
'Save Our Babies' campaign 105
scab labourers 203–4

South African Nursing Council
(SANC) 76, 78–80, 128,
146, 151, 204
control of nursing
syllabuses 142
disciplinary committee 153
identity numbers and passbooks
for nurses 146–8
South African Nursing Journal 79–80
South African Trained Nurses
Association 78
South African War 37
South Rand Hospital 109
Soweto
clinics 62–3
health care before World War
Two 31–3
health services, pre-1948 28–31
petrol bombs 203
popular resistance 164
population 31
struggle against apartheid
149–50
tourist industry 2–3
upheavals 178
uprisings 103–4
Soweto Community Council 63
Spanish influenza 29
spinal stenosis 91
squatter movement 32
stab wounds 46
to spine, heart, abdomen 91
staff morale 187
shortages 143, 165, 178, 200, 207
state funding to black hospitals 163
states of emergency 163, 164–5

state-sponsored violent
oppression 163
statistics 6, 164
St John's Ambulance 37–8
Stockdale, Sister Henrietta 37
stress in workplace 107–8
strikes 22, 125, 162, 164, 200–6
Baragwanath Hospital 152
death threats 203
and demonstrations,
nurses' 145–55
full-scale 206
intimidation and violence 203
liable for dismissal 149
peaceful demonstration 147
wage, by non-medical
workers 151–2
wildcat 206
struggle patients 101
substandard patient care 165
support groups 144
Swanson, Maynard W 14
Sweet, Helen 22

TAC, *see* Treatment Action Campaign
Tambo, Adelaide 125
Tambo, Oliver 125
'Taung child' hominid fossil 47
tax system for nurses 206
teamwork in emergency 96–7
technological care and basic
care 191
technologies as teaching tools 73
Tenza, Mpe 122, 129, 131, 133, 137,
143–4

wards
administration courses   141
sisters, black   21–2, 75
welfare policies   16
Western medicine   11
education of communities   141
and indigenous medicine   141
West Rand Administration Board   63
Williamson, Shirley   78
Wilson, Vernon   45–7, 105

Wits, *see* University of the
Witwatersrand
Witwatersrand, *see* Gauteng
work ethic, medical staff's lack
of   179
World War Two, *see* Second World
War
wounds, head, neck, abdomen   92

Zungu, Anastasia   136, 140, 143

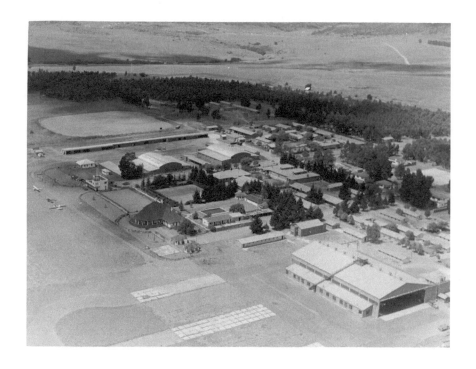

Plate 1: Early aerial photograph of Baragwanath as a military hospital.

Courtesy the author.

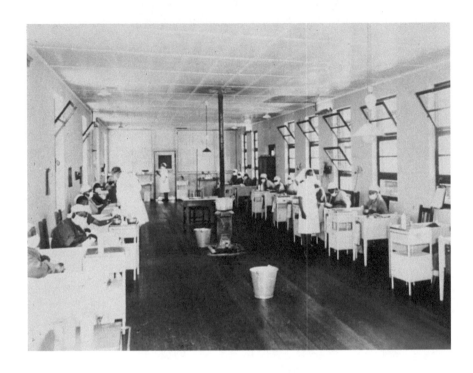

Plate 2: Premature baby unit (Ward 40) at Baragwanath Hospital in the 1950s heated by coal-fired tubular stoves.

Photograph taken by Professor Sam Wayburne.

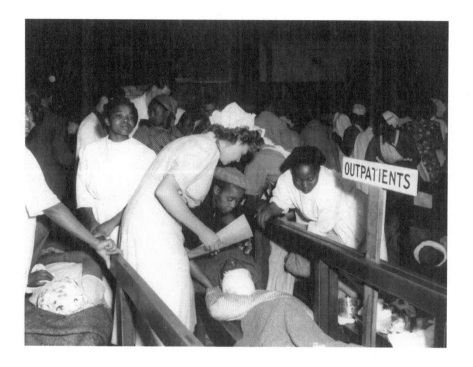

Plate 3: Outpatients ward in the 1950s.

Courtesy MuseumAfrica.

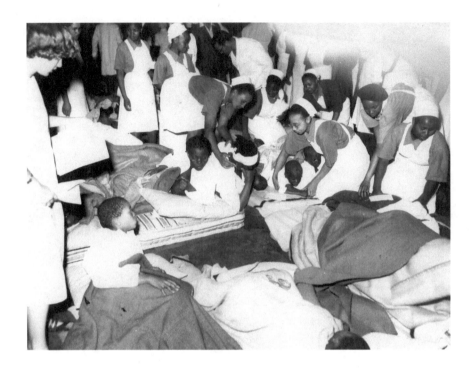

Plate 4: Patients on mattresses being tended by nurses and doctors.

Courtesy MuseumAfrica.

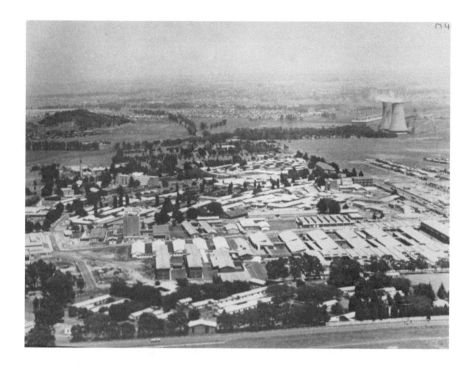

Plate 5: Aerial photograph of Baragwanath Hospital with Soweto in the background.

Courtesy the author.

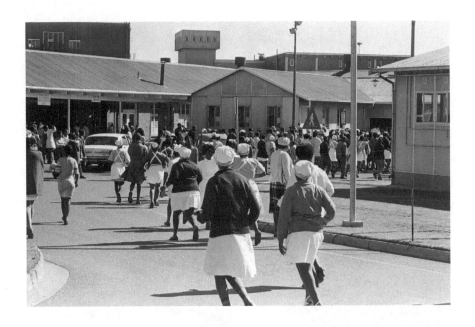

Plate 6: Nurses' strike at Baragwanath Hospital in the late 1950s

Courtesy MuseumAfrica.

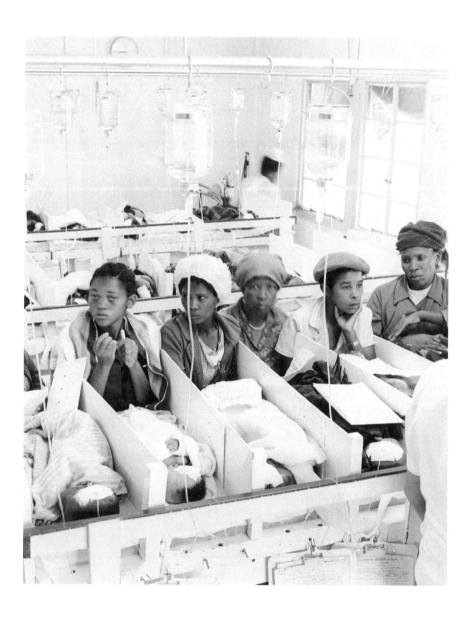

Plate 7: Mothers watching over babies on drips being treated for gastroenteritis.

Photograph by David Goldblatt.

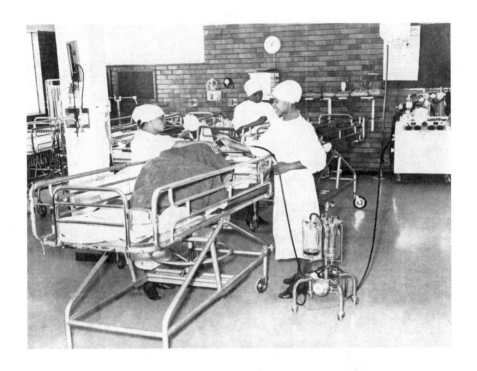

Plate 8: Nurses treating patients in post-operative care.

Photograph by Claude Provost, Panorama Magazine 1967.